Overcoming Common Problems

Letting Go of Perfectionism

YESEL YOON

sheldon PRESS

First published by Sheldon Press in 2024
An imprint of John Murray Press
A division of Hodder & Stoughton Ltd,
An Hachette UK company

2

This book is for information or educational purposes only and is not intended
to act as a substitute for medical advice or treatment. Any person with a
condition requiring medical attention should consult a qualified
medical practitioner or suitable therapist.

A CIP catalogue record for this title is available from the British Library

Library of Congress Control Number: 2024934219

Trade Paperback ISBN 9781399817318
eBook ISBN 9781399817325

Typeset by KnowledgeWorks Global Ltd.

Printed and bound in Great Britain by Clays Ltd, Elcograf S.p.A.

John Murray Press policy is to use papers that are natural, renewable and
recyclable products and made from wood grown in sustainable forests.
The logging and manufacturing processes are expected to conform to
the environmental regulations of the country of origin.

John Murray Press
Carmelite House
50 Victoria Embankment
London EC4Y 0DZ

The authorised representative in the EEA is Hachette Ireland, 8 Castlecourt Centre,
Dublin 15, D15 XTP3, Ireland (email: info@hbgi.ie)

www.sheldonpress.co.uk

Contents

*To all of the imperfect human beings who have
had the courage to share parts of themselves
and their journey with me.*

About the author

Dr. Yesel Yoon, Ph.D. is a licensed clinical psychologist and a therapist, writer, and speaker. Her specialties lie in helping people with perfectionism, identity and career exploration. In all her work, her mission is to enable others to feel more confident in their ability to re-think and re-learn old patterns and learn to be more accepting of themselves so they can live a more fulfilling life.

In her private practice she helps high achievers to overcome their struggles with perfectionism, people-pleasing, and feelings of burnout. She has presented to organizations and provided workshops and resources to help improve the mental wellbeing of their collective workplace environment. As a writer and speaker, she has contributed to various media outlets, *Psychology Today*, her website blog, and mental health panels.

Her experiences as a Korean American have shaped a lot of her thinking and approach to her work, and she hopes to inspire others to share their stories of collective struggle, exploration, and growth. She lives and works in New York City.

Introduction

There comes a time in your life when you realize your actions have consequences. You learn that what you say and how you behave have an effect on other people. You start to recognize that there is a good way to be and a bad way to be and if you want to avoid disapproval, shame, or rejection, you better live out the good way. You see that you can change how people treat you based on your behavior, your achievements, and your willingness to change yourself to fit their expectations. This cause-and-effect relationship between your behaviors and other peoples' reactions to you is the foundation where perfectionism begins.

Fast forward, and you've made it this far in life fulfilling your goals and other's expectations. Then why is there something gnawing at you, a little voice asking:

I've done everything by the book and yet why am I not happy?

Why can't I be grateful when I have so much going for me?

I used to be so motivated and driven but what does it mean if I don't want to keep this up anymore?

Why do I still feel like I'm not enough?

Is it just me? What am I doing wrong?

I'll never forget the day I was hiking through the woods in Mohonk Preserve with my then-husband close to my birthday, full on weeping.

On the surface, everything was going well for me. I had left my full time job and decided to transition into my private practice full time. I was in my early thirties, was newly married, lived near New York City, and rented an office in Midtown Manhattan. I had successfully gotten my Doctorate in Clinical Psychology by the age of 30, finished additional post doctoral training, became a licensed clinical psychologist, and was now the owner of a burgeoning practice that I'd built on my own. Things on the outside appeared to be the ideal outcome for someone like me who had taken her professional career so seriously and prided herself in being such a high achiever. My family seemed pleased with where I was in my life. I had a solid answer to the question so often asked at dinner parties, "What do you do?" and I would get nods of approval. People seemed impressed.

Then why in the world was I in tears in the middle of the woods?

How My Path Towards Perfectionism Began

My racial, gender, ability, and class identities shaped how I was raised, the kinds of values that were instilled in me, and the representations of "success" I was exposed to. I am a cisgender, non-disabled, Korean American female who was born and raised in the United States in a two-parent opposite-sex married household. Both of my parents immigrated to the U.S. from South Korea for professional and educational pursuits and raised my younger brother and me in the U.S. During my adolescent years, our family moved to the East Coast where my education and social life were embedded within a competitive, upper-middle class ethnically diverse and highly educated environment.

I had the privilege of growing up with access to resources that supported my upward academic and career trajectory. I had financial, housing, and food security so I could focus on what seemed most important - achieving financial stability and career success. It was clear that those things were revered in this world, and I had some direction on how to get those things.

As one of my Asian American clients once described, I always had this sense that I needed to "earn my keep." I did this by trying to be the "perfect" version of myself at school, at home, and in my relationships. I told my friend once that I grew up learning how to be an "expert direction-taker." This means I spent my early childhood years perfecting the art of taking directions from other people in positions of authority and delivering excellent, timely, above-and-beyond results. Because the need to stand out and prove myself started so early, it makes sense that it was only a matter of time until something broke and it was too much.

That day in the woods was just one of those painful fork-in-the-road, come-to-Jesus moments that life throws at you when it's time to learn something very real about yourself. I was facing the harsh reality that while I had done so much that appeared to bring happiness to others, I wasn't actually that happy. This scared me. I had to finally admit to myself how tired I was of chasing after the things I'd been told were symbols of being good and worthy of approval.

I've witnessed similar reckoning points for the many people I've worked with in my practice as a psychologist. By the time they come to work with me, it's because they're overwhelmed, confused, and scared by these questions and feelings about the state of their lives. As a psychologist, I've used my personal and educational experiences to help others navigate their lives in ways that make things easier for them. I help them get to a place where they aren't so hard on themselves, where they can see the good in themselves just as others can see them, and where they can allow all the parts of themselves to work in sync. Perfectionism is just one of those various parts that people feel take over their lives and over the long run, leads to more suffering than good. They want help figuring out how to regain control over the way they feel and to be freed of an unrelenting need for approval and perfection.

I do not believe in a "cure" or a "fix" for perfectionism. I make it clear at the outset to my clients that this is an unrealistic expectation. I attempted to "fix myself" by trying to out-perform, out-think, or out-feel perfectionism. I thought I could find some lifehack, read enough books, and apply the "Perfect Optimal Strategy" to fix how I was feeling. I believed this was just like any other problem in my life that I was able to overcome through sheer grit and determination. Spoiler alert, this didn't work. Instead, my constant striving for a perfect way to outdo perfectionism only made things worse.

If there's one thing I've learned through all my ups and downs, my professional training, and my work with clients, it's that you won't get very far trying to get rid of the parts that make up who you are.

This book aims not to help you cure something that you think is broken or wrong with you. This book aims to have you examine the roots of perfectionism, build more awareness of its role in your life, and learn strategies to manage how it manifests so it is working with you as opposed to against you. This book reflects what I've learned from my own experiences as a high-achiever, a people-pleaser, and a perfectionist.

I noticed that so much of the advice about how to overcome perfectionism, manage boundaries, and improve your mental well-being was coming from a White, Euro-centric perspective. Because of this, I often felt like something was missing or didn't quite fit my circumstances. For example, the challenges I was encountering with my family relationships felt more complicated so stock advice didn't help. This is why I am writing this book as an Asian American female and therapist who uses a cultural lens to inform whatever words of advice I offer to you. The intersection of aspects of your identity affects how you experience the world and how you respond to it. My voice will hopefully resonate with people who have to consider nuanced parts of their identity and cultural upbringing when they address issues like perfectionism.

I hope you will see parts of yourself in the stories I share that are based on the experiences of clients I've had the privilege of working with. The advice, exercises, and strategies offered are a collection of tools you can use to actively work on your own relationship to perfectionism. I invite you to think about how you can take action steps after you read each chapter. It is possible to live a life where your self-worth is no longer tied to old beliefs about what it means to be "good enough." Instead, you can live with greater self-acceptance and confidence to live according to your values, a life beyond perfectionism.

What to Expect

If we want to learn how to change something, we first need to know what we're dealing with. Defining terms and using examples to illustrate what those terms mean can help us understand and make meaning of our own experiences. Therefore, Chapter One will set the stage for defining what perfectionism is. Perfectionism exists in a cluster of other related issues. For example, you can't go far from a stone's throw of perfectionism without hitting up against inner criticism, expectations, imposter syndrome, or people-pleasing. Comparisons, cultural expectations, burn-out, and anxiety, will also be brought up when I discuss perfectionism in the workplace and relationships.

After we've gotten on the same page about the concepts related to perfectionism and what it looks like, we can start to get into what I'll call The Origins of Perfectionism in Chapter Two, an answer to the question "How did we get this way?" We'll take a big-picture lens look at cultural and systemic factors such as capitalism, socioeconomic status, intergenerational cultural messages, gender, and racial identity. These macro-level societal and socio-cultural factors contribute to the experience of and maintenance of perfectionism, people-pleasing, chronic stress, and burnout in us as individuals as well as our institutions and systems.

Work is a specific setting where perfectionism and especially people-pleasing tendencies rear their heads. In Chapter Three, I will talk about how these issues come up in the workplace, in particular how people tend to over-identify with their roles at work. This leads to over-functioning or under-functioning, lack of boundaries, and constant hustling for your worth. I will share strategies on how to set boundaries at work, re-think your relationship to productivity, manage imposter syndrome, and establish more realistic expectations for how work will fit in your life.

Perfectionistic tendencies also play a big part in how we engage in our relationships. We often use the umbrella term of "people pleasing" as one example of being a perfectionist in our relationships. In Chapter Four, I'll delve into more specific ways people-pleasing shows up, such as in caretaking, the fear of vulnerability and conflict, and difficulty asking for help. I'll talk about how cultural expectations play a big role in why we try to perfect ourselves in our relationships. Sometimes your values and needs won't align with others, but it is still possible to maintain good relationships while advocating for yourself. I will provide you with some advice about how to build deeper connections and allow you to care for others while still making room for your own needs to be met.

It's hard for perfectionists to make mistakes and see those as potential positive, growth-promoting experiences. Imperfection and uncertainty can be hard to tolerate if you only see them only as setbacks. Chapter 5 will be about embracing *imperfection*. I'll share some reasons we fear imperfection and some thought patterns that keep us stuck in a perfectionistic mindset. I'll talk about the benefits of embracing imperfection and how it can co-exist with enoughness. Imperfection is the foundation from which we can move through the world with more ease, humility, and curiosity. This chapter will help you respond to imperfect and uncertain situations with more flexibility by asking questions like "What else is possible?" or considering things as "fine for now" and "good enough".

Hopefully by the time you get to the final chapter, you'll see perfectionism less as an enemy that must be destroyed and "fixed", and more as a well-intentioned but overused employee whose job description needs to be re-written and reassigned. Chapter Six will help you acknowledge the adaptive role perfectionism played in your life and how it can continue to co-mingle with the other parts of you. So much of your identity gets lost when you center others' expectations and needs and spend your time and resources on achieving the "perfect" outcomes. We will explore deeper questions about how you see yourself beyond being a perfectionist and how you can embody these parts of your identity in your daily life.

When we're not so busy trying to get rid of perfectionism or letting it take over, we can focus on our values and how to live in line with what we *actually* care about. I'll share exercises to help you identify your values and translate them into specific behaviors you want to guide you instead of misguided and damaging external expectations.

Why I Wrote This for You

The reason I chose to write this book is because I want other people to see the possibility of overcoming something that is so pervasive and all-encompassing. I know how it has affected my life and so many others' lives and how hard it can feel to be. There were darker times in my life when I felt like this was just "how I was built" and I'd never escape the pressure I constantly felt. I felt as if life was always going to feel like a slog of unreachable expectations, constant striving and pervasive existential exhaustion. I'm so glad that I did not accept this as the end-all-be-all to my life.

I confronted the issues that were plaguing me. I read and listened to other people's stories and advice about how to deal with these difficult feelings. When I heard how this was affecting other people, I felt immense relief. I felt other things too, such as sadness, anger, hope, and inspiration. But the overwhelming feeling was always relief. I felt relief that I was not alone, I was not somehow broken, and that I was going to be okay. If this other person was able to have some distance from their experiences with perfectionism, chronic stress, burnout, and self-criticism, then so could I. I no longer had to accept the pervious narrative that made me feel so hopeless before - that this "just how life/I was going to be." Now I had options. Similarly, I do not want anyone else to accept that their lives will always have to feel so hard, that they are broken or nothing they do will ever be enough.

And so, I've written this book so I can offer you another possibility, another option, and another person to look to and say "Look, she's gone through something like this too so I must not be alone. I must not be broken. And I, too, will be okay."

I've listened to hundreds of people in my capacity as a therapist, from all ages and stages of life, from myriad backgrounds and experiences. There are common narratives of struggle regarding perfectionism from which I'll pull to illustrate how perfectionism shows up in all of us and how it can change. I've had the fortune of witnessing my clients release themselves from the chains of unrealistic expectations and pressure and experience change. I believe this is possible for all of us. I'm excited to see what this journey will bring you.

1

Nice to meet you, perfection

When people ask me what I do, I tell them I'm a therapist and I specialize in areas such as perfectionism, burnout, chronic stress, and anxiety. Their eyes widen with recognition. They give me a knowing look when I say the word "perfectionism."

A conversation usually starts with, "Oh yeah, I'm totally a perfectionist" and then is followed up with, "So how do I stop being a perfectionist? How do I stop caring so much?"

My attempt at an answer comes from two perspectives.

One is from that of a fellow perfectionist-in-recovery. I want to say, "Well, funny you ask, I'm still trying to figure that out . . ."

The other is from that of an experienced therapist. I explain how it's a process of understanding where perfectionism comes from, what function it serves in your life, and how what you're really trying to do is to build a more workable relationship with it so it doesn't take over your life. So I reply, "You don't ever really get 'rid' of it, but you can learn how to live with it so it's not causing you so much pain."

But I'm getting ahead of myself. It's interesting that I can use the word "perfectionism" and everyone seems to just know what it is. So what exactly are we talking about when we refer to "perfectionism"?

Defining perfectionism

Perfectionism is like many human emotions and experiences. Sometimes it's hard to name it, but you can tell when you're

1

affected by it. It's clear when it's taking over your life even if you can't put it into exact, concise words. There is such power in putting a name to emotions and other internal experiences that have such potential to control how we engage in the world. When we can wrap our minds around them, we can begin to get a sense of what to do with them.

Literal definitions of perfectionism include phrases and traits such as:

"Rejecting anything less than perfection" (Dictionary.com)

"Anything short of perfection is unacceptable" (Merriam-Webster)

Philosophical and ethical definitions call perfectionism a will towards a state of being, that of being good and moral. People who come from religious backgrounds, whether they're still observing religious practices or not, tend to hold themselves to this ethos of perfection as a form of good character and deservingness. I'll get into this more in Chapter 2 when I talk about what other cultural and social phenomena contribute to perfectionism's hold on our society.

This book defines perfectionism as *a personality trait characterized by perpetual striving towards high, often unrealistic, outcomes and being overly critical.*

Internal manifestations of perfectionist traits – how one thinks and feels about themselves – include:

- imposter syndrome
- self-criticism
- black-and-white thinking
- rumination
- comparisons to others.

External manifestations of perfectionistic traits – how one interacts with the outer world – include:

- people-pleasing
- deprioritizing oneself for the sake of others' approval
- lacking boundaries between personal and other domains of one's life.

I want to introduce you to two overarching paths perfectionism can take: overfunctioning and underfunctioning.

Forms of perfectionism: the overfunctioner and the underfunctioner

The overfunctioner: the "I can do it all" types

Gabby set her bags down on the floor next to the couch in my office. "I'm sorry I'm late. I had to put out fires at work on my way here," she said, half paying attention to me and to her phone, still standing next to the couch.

"Want to have a seat?" I asked, attempting to snap her out of the daze she was clearly in; she hadn't yet even taken off her jacket or sat down.

Finally, she sent off one more message and dropped her phone into her overstuffed work tote. She sat somewhat upright, her energy remaining abuzz from being in constant-go mode and her mind a bit distracted as she was still "on" from that day's fires.

Gabby described how her week had gone, how she had spent the whole week going into the office earlier and being the last to leave. She'd come home most days with the intent to get things done at home, like laundry, sorting through the packages she still needed to return, or maybe working out. But instead, she'd logged back onto her work computer and worked till late. Eventually she'd fallen asleep on her couch, not even making it to the bedroom.

It always took a few minutes into our sessions for Gabby to wind down and be more centered. As she continued to elaborate on her daily routine, the buzzing energy she had at the start of the session started to shift. She sat back into the couch, letting some of the weight of the day sink into her body. "I just don't feel like I can say no. I don't know if I can keep going at this pace because I feel so drained. But I don't know what else to do. If only someone could stop time. I know that's stupid because we can't get more time, but seriously, I need someone to just press pause and then I can catch up on everything. Right?"

Gabby is one of many people I've seen in my therapy practice who are constantly in go-go-go mode. They describe themselves as over-achievers, Type As, and people who constantly feel the need to be productive. My clients will be the first to admit that they're perfectionists who strive for the best and expect nothing less. They have a hard time saying no to requests because they have always managed to rise to the occasion and get things done. They thrive on the energy of being on the go.

While on the surface they're highly successful, competent, and exude a sense of accomplishment and energy, beneath all that is a thick layer of fatigue, perpetual exhaustion, and buzzing anxiety. It's not that they're truly thriving from these accomplishments, it's just that they don't know what it would be like to stop.

Meet the overfunctioner.

Overfunctioning includes things like overdoing, over-scheduling, and overcommitting. It includes lists filled with tasks and projects and perpetually "biting off more than you can chew." Often an overfunctioner will complain of feeling exhausted, like they never have enough time, and will always respond to "How are you?" with "I'm so busy" and they really mean it. They feel like they can barely catch a breath.

Overfunctioners operate from the belief that if they can just get more done, reply to more emails, and complete more projects, then things will be okay. Not only will things be okay, but they will be seen as good and worthy. They tie so much of their self-worth to the amount they are able to accomplish. Overfunctioning is one avenue by which we try to deal with the desire to be seen as "perfect" or "good enough." To be seen as a good worker, a good parent, a good *insert role here*. If we can just get that one thing done, *then* we'll be good enough.

Brené Brown calls this "hustling for your worth" (p. 23, *The Gifts of Imperfection*). It's being on the hamster wheel of performance, achievement, and proving ourselves. Unfortunately, overfunctioners have the impossible task of trying to keep up in a system with ever-present updates and advances in technology, and more things we could strive to achieve. There is no end in sight because there's always more that can be done.

In the book *Four Thousand Weeks*, Oliver Burkeman refers to the constant pursuit of getting through our to-do list as a futile attempt at "clearing the decks." He normalizes the behaviors many people engage in while trying to get to the bottom of a to-do list and feel a sense of accomplishment and closure. One of many a-ha moments I experienced while reading his book was when he simply called out: *"You've already failed."* And what he meant by this was that our constant need to "re-set" and "clear the decks" was an illusion of control perfectionists try to hold on to.

Chapter 2: Origins of perfectionism will go into more detail about the reasons why we're so drawn to this need to overfunction and prove our worth.

While there are those who overdo to get the feeling of being good enough, there are also those whose experience of the pressure to get so much done and to do so perfectly gets to be too much so that they can't take the first step at all.

The underfunctioner or chronic procrastinator

On the couch in my office, Steven looked down and put his head in his hands. "I know I said I'd apply to new jobs this week, but I didn't. Here I go again. I can't seem to get myself to do anything. I'm so unmotivated. It's always the same thing. What's the point of trying again when we both know how this is going to end up?"

This wasn't the first time Steven said this to me at the start of each therapy session. Here he was, someone who had gone to multiple high-ranking schools, scraped by to earn professional academic degrees, and was employed by a reputable research institution. But he was barely getting by. He struggled to meet deadlines. He said he'd been a chronic procrastinator since he was in middle school and nothing ever worked to get him on track.

"I know what I should do. I've always been like this. Other people know how to do things, but I've never been able to get it together. It's embarrassing – I'm in my forties and it's like I never learned how to function like a regular human being."

Steven only saw himself as a chronic procrastinating, unmotivated, lazy person. He spoke of himself as someone who couldn't do things, who would never finish what he started, and who was useless compared with other people.

I did not see him this way, nor did others who cared about him and knew him well. It was my job to help him understand that his inability to take action wasn't because he was broken, "useless," or stupid, all of the things he had told himself time and time again. I wanted him to see that the real culprits were the way he spoke to himself, the unrealistic expectations he had of himself to get things done, and the underlying fears he had about failure and success. They were collectively setting him up to fail. He needed to understand that underfunctioning was an extension of perfectionism and that his high-achieving desires were hurting him.

Underfunctioning looks like avoidance, procrastination, and constant overwhelm to the point of not doing anything at all. It can look like nothing is happening on the surface. The temptation by others who are judging an underfunctioning person is to call them lazy, unmotivated, and all of the similar words Steven was using to describe himself. But this actually misses the point.

Underneath all of that surface-level "nothingness" going on is a strong desire to accomplish things to a high standard of perfection. These high standards are the root of the procrastination. You build up so much pressure around getting things done. You overcomplicate the steps to getting started. You can't imagine ever getting to the end, so you don't even bother to start. Underfunctioning is not actually because you don't care. In fact, it's often because of caring *so* much, almost *too* much, that it leads to not taking any action.

"If I don't try at all, then I won't be disappointed." This is a common phrase I hear. Whether you're avoiding completing something you started or starting something new, you're trying to avoid feeling disappointment. But when it comes to delaying action to avoid this feeling, it's only a short-term solution. In the long run, disappointment lingers. Your initial desire to try something hasn't gone away. Now you're going to experience both the disappointment of an unfulfilled desire and the disappointment in yourself for not taking action.

This was why Steven kept saying "Here I am again, I know what I should do, but what's the point of trying? We know how this is going to play out." This wasn't the first time he'd engaged in this pattern of considering action, avoiding it, and then feeling disappointed in himself after the fact. This is a vicious cycle so many people experience and it causes a lot of pain.

But even more so than avoiding the feeling of disappointment, I believe perfectionists are going to great lengths to avoid feeling a deeper-rooted feeling: shame.

Perfectionism as a way to avoid shame

"Where perfectionism exists, shame is always lurking. In fact, shame is the birthplace of perfectionism" (Brené Brown, p. 55, *The Gifts of Imperfection*). Shame is the unbearable feeling you get when you're convinced something is wrong with you, making you unlovable and unacceptable. Perfectionists use overfunctioning or underfunctioning to avoid that shame feeling. Overfunctioning is trying to outperform shame and ensure acceptance and approval by others. Underfunctioning is trying to delay action and avoid taking risks, thus avoiding mistakes, criticism, and being on the hook for potential failure and rejection.

Underfunctioning and overfunctioning: two sides of the same coin

Perfectionism plays a role in both overfunctioning and underfunctioning. When you get to the root of both presentations, the same underlying desire to be seen as good enough and to get things perfectly exists, it just manifests differently.

Some common traits of perfectionistic types include:

- striving towards unrealistic expectations
- making comparisons
- experiencing a harsh inner critic
- focusing solely on outcomes at the expense of the process.

Unrealistic pursuits towards perfection

Let's return to the definition of perfectionism and how it includes the pursuit of "nothing short of perfection." Once, I gently reminded a client, "But remember, perfect doesn't *really* exist," and she replied almost flippantly, "Yeah yeah, but . . . I can get damn near *close*." She said this with a tone of determination as though she wanted to be the one person to achieve the impossible.

Some perfectionists treat the pursuit of perfection like a game to be won. While a rational part of themselves knows there is no such thing as perfection, there's an emotional part driving them towards it anyway. They apply life hacks, optimize their schedules, and try to manipulate their bodies and minds.

A client referred to her experience of perfectionism as the "Perfectionist's Dilemma." She described how it felt like a constant push and pull between wanting things to be just right and not knowing when and/or how to stop.

I asked her, "How do you know when you've gotten it 'right'?"

She had a few responses:

"It should feel easy."
"It should be acceptable."
"It should make people happy."
"There shouldn't be any mistakes."

Confronting the "shoulds"

What she and I came to see together were the myriad "shoulds" that were dictating how she needed things to feel and appear in her life. Shoulds have felt like the bane of my existence as well as that of so many other people I know. Shoulds encompass the many assumptions we have about what "right" and "perfection" mean.

Should-ing is a setup for feeling bad about yourself. You feel trapped by oppressive conditions when you're deep in the should spiral. To make your way out of your should spirals, you need the clarity to course-correct. Clarity helps you approach things differently when you have fewer assumptions clouding your judgment. From this place of greater clarity, you'll be able to make more intentional decisions.

How do you gain this clarity? First, acknowledge where these assumptions are coming from and what internal messages you've been holding on to about how things *should* be. After I dug deeper into what stopped Steven from acting on the things he already knew he should do, it became clearer that he had such high expectations of what "done" looked like. One of the big shoulds Steven struggled with was based on how he saw himself compared to other people.

Better than, less than: metrics and comparisons

We naturally make comparisons between ourselves and other people. It's something we do in order to judge our performance or how we should look and act, and things we should have. You've probably heard or read some variations of quotes referring to the downsides of comparing yourself to others.

"Comparison is the thief of joy."

"Don't compare your insides to someone's outsides."

Call them cliché, but they're widespread and oft-repeated phrases for a reason. People fall victim to comparisons and the negative feelings resulting from them. What's usually happening is that they're making unfair comparisons between themselves and other people. What I mean by "unfair" is that they're using an inappropriate metric for the situation at hand. For example, think of a time you took up a new hobby. Take baking. If you compare your abilities as a novice baker to those of an executive pastry chef who has 20 years of experience, that's wholly unfair. It's an inappropriate metric of comparison. It may make more sense to compare your first-time baking skills to those of another hobbyist baker, someone else who recently took up the same activity. But even then, there are so many unknown factors that contribute to a person's performance or "outsides" that you aren't accounting for.

This other hobbyist baker may have grown up in a family of bakers and was exposed to a foundation of baking knowledge that you don't have. Therefore, making comparisons leaves you vulnerable to harboring negative thoughts towards yourself and falling down a comparison rabbit hole. I don't know how often people describe their experiences by comparing themselves to positive ones.

The only exception (and this can be a useful strategy to offset the negative effects) is to make what are called downward comparisons. This is just what it sounds like – when you compare your situation to that of one that's a bit worse off or lesser than. This can be an effective way to regain perspective. For example, when you're comparing how much money you have or how many material things you own to people who have less than you, it puts into perspective how much you actually have. The point is then to be grateful for what you have and to make the most of what you have. To be clear, downward comparison is not a way to put down anyone else or get to the point of elevating yourself in any sort of holier-than-thou type of way. It's simply useful in terms of putting yourself and your circumstances in perspective.

More often than not, the negative comparisons you're making that leave you feeling worse are the upward comparisons. When you do that repeatedly and only use those unfair upward comparisons to negate your own experiences, judge and criticize yourself, it's not helpful. A positive way to use upward comparisons is to regard the person or situation to which you're comparing your own as motivation and inspiration for what is possible. For example, as a woman of color making my way through the graduate and postdoctoral stages of my psychology career, it was helpful to see other licensed clinicians and professionals of color who were making their way as tenure-track professors or private practice owners or educators in the mental health space. In this case, I compared my situation to those of people who were in a similar field but further along in their careers. This made me feel hopeful for what could be possible for me and that there were other people out there doing what I wanted to do.

There is a two-way street between perfectionism and making comparisons. It's hard to know which comes first. Do we start to have these unrealistic perfectionistic tendencies because we compare ourselves to others? Or do we compare ourselves in order to try to perfect our lives? Either way, they're cut from the same cloth – they're both examples of overly negative and critical mental patterns. The unrealistic nature of our expectations can come from comparing ourselves and using the things we're comparing ourselves to as the new metric that we need to reach in order to be "perfect" or good enough.

The inner critic: the harsh voice of perfectionism

Emily was tearful as she shared, "I feel like if I let my guard down and be kind to myself, I'll become useless and unproductive. There's this voice in my head that reminds me how I can't stop." This voice she spoke of was that of her inner critic.

The inner critic is another name for the perfectionistic voice in your head. The inner critic is a familiar foe that constantly makes negative comments and judgments about your abilities, your accomplishments, your looks, and your worthiness. The inner critic rears its head before you try something, while you're doing something, and after you've done something. As a social being who wants to feel connected and emotionally and psychologically safe, you'll go to great lengths to avoid anything that threatens this. Sometimes the way the inner critic rears its head is by convincing you that you're never enough and leading you down the path of constant striving.

The ever-moving goalpost

Too often you set a goalpost and then, before you know it, you're moving the goalpost bit by bit until you're so far from the initial goal that you set. You might wonder why things feel so tiring and frustrating no matter how hard you try. It's because you're setting yourself up with such high expectations. These expectations might have been built up from other people initially, such as parents, coaches, or teachers. But somewhere along the way, you create your own expectations and they reach limits beyond what any human being could accomplish. It's not a bad thing to want good, high-quality things from yourself. But what if it's costing you your happiness? What if just trying to get there is so miserable that you can't stop to even enjoy any part of the process, much less the reward or outcome?

Smell the roses: how to acknowledge the process

When was the last time you really let yourself relish something you were doing? Did you really give yourself credit for the things you achieved? Do you give yourself credit for showing up and putting in the effort? Why is it so hard for us to give ourselves this credit?

The saying "smell the roses" refers to the act of slowing down and noticing what is. It requires you to be present for little things, the details of life, and the achievements, no matter how big or small. As cliché as the advice is, to "enjoy the process" or "smell the roses," the advice is there for a reason. It's because when you *don't* do it, you're quite unhappy.

If you're not willing to acknowledge the things you are doing, then you're going to keep looking at the things you're not doing. It's no wonder why people feel such a sense of lack, as though they're not enough or not doing enough. Discounting what one has and what one has done is a setup for self-criticism and discouragement. It takes practice to combat this tendency to overlook your accomplishments. You can start by taking a daily inventory of the things you did, what you enjoyed, and how it felt to experience certain things in a given day.

Gabby felt as though she should know how to get it all done in the amount of time she had. She felt things would be easier once she achieved her to-do list. She thought that if she only did things better, faster, more efficiently, then she'd clear the decks.

How do we start to get out from under this burden of constant striving?

Give yourself permission to do things your way

There is so much written out there about goal-setting and making to-do lists that help you get things done. This isn't about rehashing old advice. But what I will offer here is the reminder and permission to give yourself to make things smaller, easier, and more mentally and practically manageable.

I find that it's less about knowing how to reset goals and more about the emotional permission that people have to give themselves to take a different approach towards doing things. It's less about knowing how to break down big projects into smaller, more manageable tasks and more about accepting that, by doing this, you are not failing or doing something "less than." Your approach is not less valid or less legitimate.

Perfectionism is tricky because it dictates how we are supposed to go about getting things done, including how we should set goals. The systems we put into place to live our lives don't need to be so complicated. If the point of getting things done is indeed to *get it done*, then why not make it realistic, practically approachable, and meaningful?

What does meaning have to do with goal-setting?

Meaningfulness, significance, and the experience of doing things are often lacking and deprioritized. Perfectionists tend to focus so much on the getting-it-done part and doing it "right" and "perfectly" that they forget the actual process and experiential part of it. How about the human being who is doing all of this? What is it all for anyway?

Sometimes doing a task is simply that: a task to be completed. There doesn't have to be that much meaning imbued in going through your finances, taking care of household tasks, and submitting work projects. However, there are certain experiences in our lives when it would do us a lot more good to pay attention to how we feel while we're doing them. How can you pay attention to the experiences you're going through?

First, knowing your *why, your reason*, for what you're doing can change the whole experience of it. Often, we're driven by external motivators and others' motivators but we forget about our own internal motivations.

Second, if you can be more mindful and present during the actual events themselves, you will notice so much more. Presence requires intentionality – that you will be here, not somewhere else thinking about what happened in the past or what may be in the future.

Third, going into an experience with a mindset of gratitude and openness will help you see and experience the potential benefits of something. I find that when I am going in with the mindset of "What will I learn here? What else will I get to experience that I typically wouldn't?" it helps me stay grounded in what's about to happen. Rather than constantly assessing my performance and how well I'm doing (again, orienting more towards your performance, grading yourself),

I'm just thinking, "Wow, I can't believe I'm doing this right now" or "I'm so glad I get to finally try this" or "I'm grateful I even get this opportunity to be here right now."

All of these shifts in mindset and ways of experiencing things might sound simple, but they require practice. They're not how many of us are oriented to think or see things. Especially for people who are biased towards performance and constant evaluation, it's hard to pivot attention to the process, not just the outcome.

These strategies are helpful in offsetting the shoulds of perfection, attempting unrealistic and constantly moving goals, and indulging in tendencies towards self-criticism. Think about what areas of your life and in what kinds of experiences you could practice these shifts in mindset and reflect on them actively – writing or talking it out.

Strategies to start working with perfectionism

1 Be realistic with yourself when it comes to your goals as well as your process. Create and use systems that work *with* you. Stop trying to be like someone else or do things the way others do it. Take into account your strengths and ask yourself what's going to best support your weaker areas. Remember not to compare what is realistic for other people. The point is to focus on what is realistic and manageable, workable, for *you*. If the point is for you to experience something and get something done, then you need to have it work *with* you as opposed to working against you.

2 Give yourself credit for what you do, from the smallest of small action steps to the bigger ones. Small steps are required in order to take anything bigger and to move anywhere. Stop diminishing your accomplishments. If you don't start practicing giving yourself credit for the things

you do, you'll always feel like shit for "never having gotten something done." Essentially, you're throwing away worthy accomplishments simply in the name of them not being "big" or "perfect" enough. That's just being mean to yourself. Tough love: stop doing that. Start collecting those wins and letting every bit count. These wins build momentum. You're proving to yourself "I can do this" and that will propel you forward as opposed to staying still or moving backwards.

3 Rely on others for help. This is similar to making things easier for yourself, whether it's simplifying your lists, steps, systems, etc., you can ask others for help. Others can include people close to you such as friends or family, but can also include coaches, therapists, assistants, teachers, or any professional whose job it is to make things easier for you. There are some people who know more about something than you do and can probably get it done in less time, more efficiently, and better than you. Move your pride aside and let someone else come in and help you.

4 Let go of old experiences and whatever stories you've been telling yourself about your abilities and worthiness. I find that perfectionists hold on very tightly to stories about what they should do, and they also hold on to stories about what they can't do because of things that happened in the past. While those stories can sometimes be helpful in us learning something, you know those cases when those stories are only holding you back. It's time to let go of things that are burdening you and weighing you down. Release those and rewrite them. Retell yourself a story that's imbued with a sense of self-forgiveness, optimism, and hope for what is to come.

These are all helpful strategies that assume your personal responsibility over the way you plan, execute, and treat yourself in the process. But what if it's much larger than outside of just what we as individuals can do? How did we get to this point of thinking we needed to hustle so hard for our worthiness? From the superficial level to the bigger life milestones, there is a non-exhaustive list of things we are supposed to have to be "living our best life." But whose life is it we're striving to live? And who defined our pictures of success? Next let's talk more about some bigger-picture factors that contribute to where perfectionism comes from.

2
Origins of perfectionism

Introduction

When I first met with Esther, she described how empty she felt despite having "done it all." She had achieved a six-figure salary before her mid thirties, graduated with honors from college, attended a prestigious MBA program, and was now in a managerial position in a financial consulting company. She could afford to live in a luxury apartment building in Manhattan. Her parents often bragged about her to their friends at home, name-dropping the title of her company and mentioning the highlight reels of Esther's life.

"This is how things were supposed to turn out," she said.

I asked her, "Then why does it look like someone just shared a piece of really bad news?"

Tears welled up as she admitted, "I feel like I did everything I was supposed to do. I should be grateful. But I'm not happy. I don't think I'm living my life. Where did I go wrong?"

What went wrong in Esther's situation wasn't because of something she didn't do "right." In fact, she had done it all correctly, according to her family and society at large. But it didn't make her happy. She was placing the blame on the wrong source.

How did we get this way? Why have so many of us internalized this narrative of perfection, striving, and performance as an ideal outcome? We've spent some time talking about what it looks like to be a perfectionist, whether it's trying to prove yourself by overdoing things or avoiding taking steps towards something because of a fear of failure. Where does this need to be "good enough" and striving come from? Why is it so pervasive? I don't think anyone would choose to be this way if they could. I certainly wouldn't.

We need to know where perfectionism's roots originate. When we do, we can manage the outgrowths from those roots – the constant striving, comparison-making, people-pleasing, and self-criticism. We can make more informed decisions about whether or not we want certain habits and behaviors to continue to exist. This chapter will introduce the broader cultural and societal roots of perfectionism. This will help us see how we started to internalize messages about what defines "success." Having a greater awareness of how outside factors have contributed to how we behave and think will allow us to be more critical and start to question what we've been taught about our worthiness.

The roots of perfectionism

We are embedded within a larger context of cultural and societal voices, values, and messages. You can imagine yourself as existing in the center of a circular diagram that has a core and layers of concentric circles around that core (see Figure 2.1).

You are at the center of this circle, at the core. Alongside you are the people closest to you with whom you interact on a daily or semi-regular basis. Depending on what period of life you're in, the individuals who make up that inner circle will change. Typically, this inner circle includes our family members, romantic partners, friends, coworkers, or teachers since most of us spend our time at home, school, or work. These individuals may be people we look up to, respect, and rely on for our sense of belonging and worthiness.

The next layer enclosing the core and inner circle includes our communities and the values of those communities. This

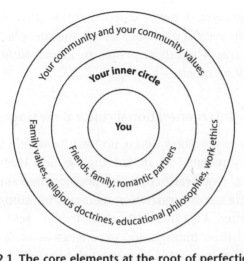

Figure 2.1 The core elements at the root of perfectionism

layer includes intergenerational family traditions and values, religious doctrines, and educational philosophies. These teach us about acceptable behavior and how we should engage with the world to be successful members of society.

Messages that fuel perfectionism are taught directly and indirectly from these systems. For example, I grew up in a highly competitive environment where I witnessed what it took to build upward social mobility. There, I learned that you should prioritize high academic and career performance, regardless of its cost to your mental and emotional well-being.

When we're younger, we don't necessarily know how to sift through the various voices that we're listening to and the messages being projected onto us. Most of us are quite vulnerable to internalizing messages that seem good on the surface. When we're told how we should be, what is right versus wrong, we're apt to take it in and listen. I was a people-pleaser and peacemaker. I never dared question the messages and instructions passed on to me from other people. This can be especially true when those people are elders, authority figures, and family members.

Intergenerational cultural messages

The types of messages I grew up hearing were a larger reflection of my parents' Asian upbringings and their immigrant experience. I've heard countless people share similar experiences as the second-generation members of immigrant households. Esther, a Chinese-American female, said her parents often used their immigration experience as evidence of their sacrifice. They reminded her repeatedly that she was supposed to be studying and practicing to improve herself and make their hard work "worth it." Every time they reminded her of their sacrifice to provide her with better opportunities, she was riddled with guilt. It's not hard to see where the need to prove and build up the portfolio of societally-ascribed achievements came from for both me and Esther. These intergenerational cultural messages added to our sense of "owing" it to those before us because of the sacrifices they made to afford the resources we had now.

Another outgrowth of the cultural roots of perfectionism is overfunctioning and an achievement-oriented mindset. Unfortunately, most of our educational systems prioritize grades, degrees, and accolades. Productivity is a measure of your worth and how far you'll get in life. You strive for anything that builds up your college application, then anything that adds to an impressive résumé, then anything that will put you on track for promotion, and so on. Rather than considering "What interests me?" or "What am I good at?," we're conditioned to think, "What will look good to so-and-so?" or "What will get me to the next stage of my career?"

People-pleasers and those who fear conflict were often told they shouldn't speak up, shouldn't "rock the boat," should show respect. This comes in the form of familial and other community values of selflessness and humility. For those of us who grew up in a religious household, "good, moral, right" behaviors are usually conditioned along those same lines.

"Doing life right"

We constantly strive for perfection, control, and to do things "right" to avoid the dreaded outcome of being judged as bad. In my journey towards unpacking the cultural roots of perfectionism, I realized that I had internalized a certain religious teaching or philosophy about what it meant to be "good." My memories of these teachings revolved around how to be a good person who was deserving of good things and eventually would have a good outcome at the end of life. "Obsession" might seem a little strong, but I truly feel that, at times in my life, I was obsessed with this need to be "doing life right." Despite the fact I'm no longer religiously observant, I haven't completely shaken myself free of this abstract fear of being found out as an unworthy, undeserving, "bad" person. I wonder, with all I was given – my abilities, resources, opportunities, and time – did I make the most of my life? Did I make the right choices? Was I a good person?

Some may call it irrational, but this is a common human existential dilemma. Not everyone's dilemma is rooted in religious teachings, but many of my clients reckon with similar questions and these questions are also drivers of their perfectionism. As Oliver Burkeman writes in *Four Thousand Weeks*, "It's not just that this situation feels impossible; in strictly logical terms, it really is impossible." This captures the same existential fears that drive our constant obsession with productivity and trying to manage our time. He brings to light the deeply rooted desire for us to be living life "right."

When you say you want to "do well," "succeed," and "do life right," what does that mean? Question what you're striving for and where it's coming from. Why are you aiming for these things? We'll delve deeper into these questions later in the book. I'll discuss how we can make values-aligned choices in our lives that aren't rooted in old cultural messages and fears. But for now, pause and give yourself a reprieve from any pressure you may be feeling. Get curious. See the connections between cultural messages you've internalized and how they've been driving your perfectionistic tendencies.

The societal roots of perfectionism

Remember those contextual layers I mentioned that we're embedded in? Now let's turn to the outermost layer, which includes societal ideologies and economic influences. Political and global events, technological trends, and societal attitudes about populations of people are included in this larger social layer of influence. Socially defined groups have vastly different lived experiences of trying to make it in the world because of racism, classism, ableism, and sexism, to name a few.

What does all of this have to do with perfectionism? Perfectionism shows up for people differently based on their value in society. These social and cultural layers show how much influence lies above and beyond the individual thoughts and feelings we have in our little brains. For instance, many people blame themselves for the negative impacts of perfectionism in their lives, even though the dominant cultural ideology of individualism encourages perfectionist tendencies. We can also refer to it as the bootstrapping mentality.

Cultural messages about achievement are so centered on individual behaviors and "work ethic." This prioritizes self and individualism in the execution of achievement as well as the onus on the self if things feel hard or don't work out. People who ascribe their self-worth to what they can achieve on their own resist asking for help, and they tend to be overly critical of themselves and other people. They place an immense amount of pressure on themselves to achieve and then blame themselves or others for mistakes. Because if it's all on us alone to succeed, then it's all on us alone when we fail. This is short-sighted and damaging. This sets us up in a warring relationship with ourselves. It's time we question these overly simplistic and harmful messages about individualism, self-reliance, and how it's our fault for feeling this way.

Societal expectations of enoughness

We see projections of what "hustling" and "living the good life" look like through channels such as the diet and wellness industry, the beauty and home improvement industry, social media, marketing, and entertainment. "Ideal" versions of what we should have, look like, and strive for bombard us constantly because systems and institutions profit when we feel we're lacking something. Under capitalism, companies and institutions drive most of our consumption and spending behaviors. The more they can make us feel we need to have more, the more we will invest our resources – including time, money, and emotional energy – into procuring those things by whatever means necessary.

The diet, "health and wellness," beauty, and related commercial industries all profit from our need to be desirable, to be approved of, and to make up for a sense of lack. There has been a lot written about the negative impact of social media and advertising on people's mental health. There's a reason we feel worse about ourselves after we look at media representations of people "living their best lives."

Perfectionistic tendencies increase in the face of these external messages that tell us we're not good enough unless we perform better, look better, and achieve more. We have to buy this or that, we have to complete and accomplish such and such a milestone – buying a home, getting a high-paying job, making a certain amount of money to afford a lifestyle worthy of praise and admiration – and then we'll be enough. There's always more we could have, and especially in our industrialized society, it doesn't seem to end in terms of availability of options.

In the short term, we may reap the benefits of what we buy or what we produce (making more money, for example). But in the long run, the systems that truly profit and gain from our investments are larger industries. We ride this wave of feeling good in the short term with feeling like we've "made it" only to be hit with another wave of "But wait! There's more!" and on it goes.

Social media has a bad reputation because of the proliferation of these marketed messages. It contributes a lot to that fear of missing out (FOMO) phenomenon. What can start as simply a distraction with some pretty images or reviews of products can quickly become a rabbit hole of questioning whether you should have better or more things. You lose sight of what will actually add value to your life and instead depend on the quick jolts of satisfaction that make you feel like you're "keeping up" and "fitting in."

Who can keep up and fit in largely depends on social status, which is determined by a variety of factors, such as race, gender, socioeconomic status, ability (mental and physical), and identity. People of color, poor, uneducated, disabled, and queer folk have much less security, safety, and societal levels of agency. Because of this disparity in social and economic rights and privileges, members of these marginalized groups often have to take it upon themselves to make ends meet and get to a baseline level of existence, much less get ahead. They overmonitor themselves and don't speak up or advocate for themselves out of fear of retaliation (e.g. being fired, harassed, and cut off from resources in their community). When people are constantly in survival mode, they feel they have to overwork and achieve higher standards to prove their place in the world. The game is set up to have them work harder and never stop. Therefore, for marginalized folks, perfectionistic tendencies towards overfunctioning and people-pleasing are supercharged not just with wanting approval but needing to survive and avoid negative outcomes.

"Death by a thousand cuts": negative consequences of toxic social and cultural messages

When you're told in so many ways that you have to be someone different and always strive for more, it takes a toll on your mental, emotional, and physical well-being. This can result in:

- substance addictions
- disordered eating
- over-exercising
- chronic stress and burnout
- severe anxiety
- mood disorders.

The above are just a few examples of the negative consequences of pervasive toxic social and cultural messages. Even if they don't meet the criteria for a diagnosable psychiatric disorder, persistent feelings of insecurity, low self-esteem, and low self-worth are issues we still need to take seriously. When larger systems and industries gain power and grow in profit, our bodies, minds, and relationships suffer the casualties. Even if you haven't personally experienced these kinds of issues, you may know of someone who has. We must be aware of how this impacts not just us but those around us. We're all affected by these messages of "you're not enough" and "you must keep striving at all costs" that are in the air we breathe. When we buy into these messages, we also hold others to the same unrealistic standards. It might not be intentional, but the biases we internalize affect the way we treat other people too.

We're mentally, emotionally, and physically compromised when we start to believe these messages of not being enough and having to attain unrealistic standards of goodness and worthiness. We adopt certain mindsets, such as a scarcity mindset and "if . . . then" thinking. These lead to behaviors such as numbing out difficult emotions, overcontrolling, and striving for self-improvement or self-optimization.

The scarcity mindset

The scarcity mindset is when we think and feel as though we don't have enough. It makes us engage in a kind of mental and psychological hoarding. Sometimes, we even engage in the literal hoarding of financial and material resources, which stems from the same sense of scarcity.

> Vicki reached financial independence in her midthirties, a goal she set from the time she left her childhood home. She grew up in a household where both emotional and financial resources were scarce. She didn't receive much positive attention or affection from her immediate family members and her parents reminded her that if she wanted something, she'd have to figure out how to get it herself. Now, as an adult, she had a bank account reflecting to her that she had indeed "figured it out." Rationally, she knew she was free to make more liberal spending decisions and life

choices. She could leave her job today if she wanted. However, she felt the need to continue working 60–80-hour weeks. She continued to save every last dollar, denying herself takeout meals or outsourcing any tasks in her life.

I asked her why she continued to save despite having enough.

She replied, "It still doesn't feel like enough. Other people continue to work just as hard or harder than me, so if I stop, then I might fall behind. I'm afraid if I don't work as hard, then I won't be able to provide and no one will take care of me."

Her savings and lack of spending, her desire to continue accumulating more resources despite what she possessed, were all manifestations of trying to gain a semblance of security.

When others tell us we're one step away from failing or losing it all, we develop a scarcity mindset. At the end of the day, we want to feel secure and safe, and we'll go to any means necessary to achieve those feelings. It's not wrong to want peace of mind that you and your loved ones are taken care of, but often we're considering the wrong sources of security based on the message we receive from others and society about what may fulfill that need. Enoughness is what we're all striving for and society gives us false solutions for that sense of enoughness. It's something we need to watch out for and we also need to beware of falling into the "if . . . then" trap.

The trap of "if . . . then" thinking

It may not be hard for you to think of examples of "if . . . then" thinking:

- If I lose weight, then I'll be desirable.
- If I get that promotion, then I'll be secure.
- If I save up this much money and put off spending on myself, then I'll be that much closer to freedom.
- If I stay quiet and don't make a fuss, then people will accept me.

My clients tell me that they'll start taking better care of themselves after they've finished making progress on their career goals. Or they tell me how they need to prioritize other people's needs before they can consider taking a break, attending to themselves, or asking for help. "If . . . then" thinking often results in putting off our own needs for joy and rest. This leads to burnout and resentment when we're perpetually deferring our lives for the sake of fulfilling other people's expectations.

Coping mechanisms: numbing and controlling

When we feel we don't have enough, we seek quick fixes to make those feelings of insecurity and low self-worth go away. This includes numbing through substance use, shopping, mindlessly using social media platforms, or other unhelpful behaviors.

> One of my clients, Alyssa, described how she would use Instagram to put out a version of herself to the public that appeared to "have it all" while internally she struggled to feel desirable or worthy of connection. She stuck to interacting with social media followers but didn't want to meet people in real life. She was afraid if people saw her for who she "really was," they wouldn't accept her.
>
> Alyssa's time on Instagram also provided entertainment as she observed other people's "best lives." She spent hours looking at people on her feed to feel like she was connected to a better life. This was a kind of numbing behavior that allowed her to avoid looking at her own life and confronting her feelings of insecurity and loneliness.

An alternative to numbing is overcontrolling. As a way to cope with the feelings of overwhelm and insecurity, some people double down on following rules and rituals. They use restrictive and rigid behaviors to perform external control while otherwise feeling a lack of internal control or stability. This often comes up in the form of disordered eating and over-exerting one's body and mind through work, caretaking, or exercise. Some of the most disciplined and perfectionistic people have this immense need for control; at some point in their lives, it became a coping mechanism and then they were often rewarded for appearing to have it all together. Society reinforces these addictive and controlling behaviors since it leads people to do more and produce more for others. This is where we also see the need for continual self-improvement, constant optimization, and high performance.

Constant pursuit of self-improvement and optimization

Perfectionists describe themselves as high achievers, strivers, status-driven, and very "accomplished" types. They have been "successful" in many senses of the word. Scarcity mindset and perfectionism go hand in hand, which leads to this constant desire to self-improve and optimize aspects of our lives. There isn't something inherently wrong with wanting to grow, change, and "be better." But I want you to be honest about how much it takes over your emotions and the decisions you make about how you spend your time. It's one thing to want change and a sense of accomplishment, which are very human and adaptive feelings. It's another to have it be a persistent, unrelenting, fear-driven approach to your life. "Approach" assumes there's some intentionality and mindful awareness behind your behaviors. Often, this is not the case. Instead, people operate their lives on a default setting towards striving fueled by a sense of never-enoughness and keep pursuing more/better/different without stopping to question why or what for.

It's time to break out of this default setting and recognize you have other options. I've covered some of the societal and cultural messages that contribute to our need to strive, optimize, and work for our sense of worthiness. It can feel daunting and demoralizing to realize how so much toxic cultural messaging has cost you in terms of your mental, emotional, and physical health. When I became more educated about the societal-level factors influencing how I and my clients were feeling, I became angry. That anger led me to start making more intentional choices. I felt empowered to find answers to the question: What can we do about it?

How to deal with the cultural and societal noise

I say to a lot of my clients, "It's not your fault, but it is your responsibility." In other words, we can do something about this. It is easy to fall into a pit of despair when you realize there are larger forces out there scheming to undermine your sense of self-worth to make a buck (or millions). But I challenge you to have hope and remember:

You are not alone.

You and I have the agency and power to choose how to invest our resources in what is meaningful to us.

We must reach out to one another for support and work collectively to be well.

We can deal with this by exposing ourselves to counter-cultural messaging and a breadth of diverse representations of how a person can exist in the world. We can immerse ourselves in spaces where we are taught how to live human-centered and community-oriented lives. We don't have to keep investing time and resources into systems that don't have our well-being in mind. We can limit the exposure we have to objectifying and materialistic messages. We can ask critical questions and be more discerning about the messages we see and hear, and what we choose to internalize and live out daily.

Here is a list of specific things you can do:

1 Build self-awareness and take inventory of your current social and cultural sources of influence.

   - Take an inventory of your time and money investments: where are your money, time, and attention going? You'll be surprised by how much gets taken up by things that don't add much value. You can ask why you've continued to spend your resources there and whether it's still worth that investment.

   - Take an inventory of your inner circle: who are the people you surround yourself with on a daily and regular basis? What are their values? You can tell a lot based on how they choose to spend their time, and resources, and what they might talk about a lot. Do their values align with yours? Think about how these people's values and life decisions may be influencing you both positively and negatively.

   - Take an inventory of your outer circle of social/cultural media exposures: look at the social media accounts you follow on various platforms. There is a ton of noise out there and you need to be deliberate about the volume and content of that noise. Who are the people you look at, listen to, and read? Question why you're still following them and what you get out of doing so. How do you feel after you've spent some time with their content? If it leaves you feeling worse about yourself, wasting more time than you intended, or making comparisons and falling into the scarcity mindset, then consider un-following/un-subscribing, basically blocking yourself from those accounts. You can cut off the source of toxic and useless noise. You don't have to expose yourself to people and messages that contribute to a sense of lack.

- This act of paying attention and taking inventory is powerful because you're applying mindfulness to what can often become mindless, default behaviors, and things you've taken for granted. Once you're more aware of these behaviors, you can start to make better, more informed decisions. This can help you stop resorting to default perfectionistic mindsets and behaviors.

2 Redefine what success means to you.

- Return to the shoulds we discussed in the last chapter. The shoulds include how things need to look and feel if we are to consider ourselves "doing life right." For example, when you think of someone who is "successful," who do you think of? What comes to mind as markers of "success"? You may have a certain profile of achievements and expectations not unlike what my client described as how she was "supposed to" turn out.

- What has it meant to be "successful" or "good enough"? Are your current beliefs about these terms based on your own beliefs or those of someone else? Where did those messages come from? This may be related to the answers above when you took inventory of your inner and outer circles.

- Write a new definition by describing what "being well" (not "doing well") looks and feels like. Get creative and don't limit yourself. Don't worry about what you think should be in your new description and definition.

3 Expose yourself to counter-cultural messages.

- Find diverse representations of how a person can exist in the world. Find a range of bodies, lifestyles, careers and upbringings, identities, political and social views. You were previously exposing yourself to quite a limited subset of messages and personalities, so now is when you get to discover new and different avenues of expression.

There are so many directions you can go in, the possibilities are endless, and that's the fun and hopeful part of this!

- Immerse yourself in spaces where you hear and see people who uplift the more person- and community-centered approach to living as opposed to objectifying and materialistic messages.
- When it comes to divesting from certain relationships, it's not as simple as cutting people off, especially family members. It isn't sound or culturally sensitive advice to tell someone to stop associating with or "just stop caring" about certain people and certain messages. There are cultural values of loyalty and who is considered "family" which make it more complicated. I'll go into this more in Chapter 4 about perfectionism in relationships.

4 Become a more critical and conscious consumer.
- Divest your time and resources from industries that don't have your best interest in mind.
- Spend less money on things and more on experiences.
- See where in your life you can afford to spend more time and attention. This can take the shape of healing your relationship with your body, exercise, healthy relationships, pleasure, leisure, and rest.

5 Practice the inner work of self-reflection and reframing your thoughts and beliefs. Often we're pursuing fixes, perpetual growth, and optimization because we're avoiding a feeling or have trouble accepting what is. Ask yourself:
- Where is the need to fix, optimize or "grow" coming from? Is it coming from a sense of lack and perpetually needing to fix and change myself?
- What is stopping you from feeling okay with what is? What about yourself or your current circumstances is hard to accept and why might it be difficult to accept?

- Are you trying to escape or avoid a sense of lack and
  unworthiness? Are you trying to be better than a version
  of yourself or someone else?

It's never too late

Maya Angelou once said:

> I did then what I knew how to do. Now that I know better,
> I do better.

I love this quote because it helps me feel empowered to make
a change once I've learned something new about myself. As
a perfectionist, I can get discouraged when I feel I got something wrong, including buying into unhelpful ways of thinking about a situation. Angelou's quote reminds me to lean
into self-compassion so that I can move forward with a more
hopeful attitude as opposed to a critical one.

All of these ways of re-engaging with the world are acts
of self-protection and empowerment. Unless someone challenges us with a different perspective, we don't question the
thoughts and feelings we have or second-guess the things
we do. They've become habitual or fit in with what we see
around us. But once we learn there are other options for how
to engage with the world, it helps us see things differently.
Rethinking things can help us make more conscious choices.

Whether you're choosing to unfollow a social media account
or choosing new ways of spending your time and money, you
don't have to go through changes alone. Share your takeaways
from this chapter with someone else. We can offer this new
perspective to other people and perhaps they, too, will change
how they think and how they invest their time and resources.

Much later in my life when I was given permission by other
people, social activists, therapists, and friends, I began my personal work of undoing the toxic messages I had internalized

for so long. To be honest, it sometimes overwhelmed me and it led me to feel a lot of anger and sadness. I thought, "How come no one else told me that I didn't have to live like this? How come I've been operating from these prescribed rules that don't really apply to me?"

It's okay to start questioning some of the assumptions and the shoulds that were ascribed to you. Hopefully, this information will stop you from placing so much blame on yourself for constantly feeling overwhelmed, burned out, or insecure. Remember, the reasons we have felt this way have less to do with individual choices we've made and rather more to do with the larger systemic, societal, and cultural forces around us.

Now that you know better, you can do better for yourself and others around you. It's never too late to unlearn old messages and relearn new ones that help improve the quality of your life and not have this sense of not-enoughness steer you towards those perfectionist tendencies that do more harm than good.

3
Perfectionism at work

Introduction

Work is a domain where perfectionism runs rampant. Workplaces require people to deliver results in exchange for higher salaries and benefits, promotions, verbal and written validation, and evaluations. One of the various traps in this kind of work-for-rewards environment is that often you can lose sight of what is realistic in terms of the resources you need and time you require to constantly deliver. I don't think it's a coincidence that we often hear the words "work" and "never ending" together. People have a hard time knowing how much to take on and can easily get overwhelmed. The two paths people take are either to attempt to do it all (i.e. overfunctioning) or to simply avoid it and try to get the least amount done because it all seems too daunting (i.e. underfunctioning.)

At work, you can quickly start to feel as though you're only aiming for people's approval and to survive the work environment, not necessarily that you're working for quality or contributing to anything meaningful. The combination of constant delivery and reduced meaning in your output leads to negative feelings about your effectiveness – in other words, burnout. I'll go into greater depth about how we're influenced by toxic work culture and societal messages about what is deemed "productive" and markers of "success."

Early work memories: how we learn to value work

In order to build a healthier relationship to work we need to understand where we're starting from. It is important to see how we came to associate work with our self-worth and why we carry certain emotions and expectations about the role work plays in our lives. We can do this by reflecting on our earlier work memories and the messages we internalized from those experiences.

When I was a child, my mother would buy workbooks at a teaching supply store (mind you, she's not a teacher, I don't know how she even thought of this option) so that we'd keep up our studies during summer breaks on top of our time at day camp, church, Bible school, and family vacations. Every summer, our daily schedules dictated how many pages we should get done. My takeaways from this yearly practice were:

1 Academic excellence and constantly learning were keys to success.
2 Doing these academic and work-related activities were keys to winning people's approval.
3 There are productive and non-productive ways to use your time.

Unsurprisingly, I quickly caught on that productive uses of time were the better option of the two.

My parents valued a good education and a good work ethic. It was never a question of whether I'd get an undergraduate degree but rather a matter of how I'd increase my chances of getting into a good school. This meant I needed to prioritize achieving good grades and participate in the right kinds of activities that could help me in this pursuit.

These cultural messages and experiences shaped my relationship with productivity, high achievement, and prioritizing academic and work achievements above other domains of my life. I made tradeoffs in my personal life to make strides in my professional life.

Many clients I've worked with have walked similar roads with similar sounding upbringings. While this serves us well for the society we live in, making too many tradeoffs can become detrimental to our overall well-being and happiness later down the road.

Examining your work-related memories and messages

Take some time to reflect on the following questions about your experiences with work, starting from an early age. Keep these notes handy as we'll return to them and add more thoughts throughout the chapter.

1 What are some of your key academic/work-related memories? When can you first remember being aware that work mattered?
2 Were these positive, negative, or neutral experiences?
3 Based on those memories, what were some key lessons you took away? What are messages you internalized as a result of these experiences?

Work archetypes for perfectionists

We can apply the same framework of overfunctioning and underfunctioning as two general categories of perfectionistic behaviors when it comes to work. Examples of over- and underfunctioning at work include:

• overcommitting and taking on more work than is necessary or realistic

- chronic procrastination and avoiding work
- imposter syndrome and fear of being "found out" as a failure or fraud
- lacking separation between work and personal life and work taking over your life despite your desire to "shut off"
- overly identifying with the job you have and deriving your sense of worth and self-esteem from your job
- feelings of burnout and exhaustion due to a lack of boundaries and losing a sense of effectiveness or purpose at work.

In addition to the overfunctioner and the underfunctioner, later on we will cover the imposter and the workaholic.

The overfunctioner

Workplace expectations and our culture's over-emphasis on productivity contribute to a tendency towards overdoing at our jobs. Your job requires you to perform and function at the highest level and to many different levels and people. Whether you personally identify as one or you work for one, you may recognize the following signs of the overfunctioner at work:

- They tend to agree to almost anything that is presented to them.
- They don't delegate or take things off their list of responsibilities despite taking on more.
- They overpromise on the number of things they can deliver as well as the timeline of when they can get things done.
- They don't account for the increased workload in the general landscape of their lives, so outside of work they are at max capacity.

Overfunctioners are at high risk of going beyond their maximum capacity and in fact may reach it multiple times a day, week, or month. Take a moment to consider the last time you pushed yourself beyond your physical, emotional, and mental capacity at work. How did you know that you had surpassed your limits? Perhaps you felt physically exhausted, mentally fatigued, and emotionally drained. Often, you'll hear people describe feeling "burned out" due to their job and trying to balance work with the other responsibilities in their lives.

The relationship between boundaries and work-related burnout

Work-related burnout often stems from difficulty with asserting boundaries. Establishing boundaries encompasses saying no to requests, delegating, advocating for certain work conditions, and separating personal and work lives. This difficulty comes from people's fear of negative consequences such as disappointing others, getting fired or mistreated, and not attaining the positive rewards promised if they comply with what's being asked of them. "Perfect" behavior at work is a way to maintain a semblance of security (again, this is culturally and socially dependent behavior).

Kai was fed up with being treated like a "pushover." In my office, she confessed, "I feel like I'm punished for being good at my job. It's like the more I do, the more I'm asked to do. It never stops."

"What would it be like to say no to some of these requests?" I asked.

She looked at me with horror. "Oh, no! I can't imagine that would go well. These people rely on me. I can't let them down."

But time passed and the more work she did, the more requests came in. Kai felt the pressure of the internalized expectation that she must constantly be doing and delivering on promises to her colleagues.

One day, she came to our session angrier than I'd ever seen her. Earlier, she just found out several of her colleagues had been promoted and she hadn't. She'd hit her breaking point. "When will I get the recognition for the stuff I'm doing?" she exclaimed. "What is all of this for?"

In Kai's case, the perfectionistic traits of doing things so well worked against her. Because the workplace could take advantage of these skills while she didn't necessarily speak up for what she needed, she reached the point of burnout.

This situation comes from a sheer lack of practice with speaking up for what you need and want. Therefore, one of the strategies to combat this is to start doing it more often. This can be done in lower-stakes situations to build up that self-advocacy, boundary-setting muscle.

The importance of owning your voice

Owning your rightful place in the workplace and getting the treatment you deserve requires practice in asserting your voice and speaking up for what you need. This also means you need to stop qualifying the things you say. What do I mean by "qualifying" things?

- "Not that I am saying . . ."
- "I don't mean to bother you but . . ."
- "I'm sorry, but . . ."
- "I'm not sure . . ."

The need to qualify your statements comes from trying to say things "perfectly" so you don't offend someone or get criticized. People want to avoid any blow back for having a point of view that not everyone might agree with.

Kai spoke of how she "absorbed everything." She recognized that her fear of confrontation came from a childhood during which she was told to "put [her] head down." She came to believe that if she spoke up, she'd make other people uncomfortable and then she'd be punished. This could mean people wouldn't like her and she would make problems worse for herself and for others.

Societal expectations, stereotypes, and socialization (gender, race) contribute to the varying degrees in which people engage and communicate with each other. For example, women tend to qualify their statements more than men. People of color have to be especially careful about what they say and how they say things to avoid confirming stereotypes or being seen as "too angry, aggressive," somehow threatening to the listener. Similarly, those who experience imposter syndrome struggle to speak up because they feel vulnerable to getting "found out" as the imposter they believe themselves to be.

Instead, you need to own what you have to say, own your voice, and assert your power within the workplace as much as you can. You have to accept the fact that not everyone will like you or what you have to say. I understand that for people-pleasers and perfectionists, that is a difficult pill to swallow!

However, if we're constantly minimizing ourselves in order to fit in and get by in work spaces where we spend so much of our mental energy and physical resources, we're not going to make it very far. From a psychological and physical level, it'll be hard to maintain your sense of well-being. Professionally speaking, you'll be compromising yourself with these series of qualifying and personal minimizations.

Just to be clear, minimizing and qualifying can be a strategic move. In order to feel psychologically safe in the workplace, sometimes you have to adopt these communication styles. But this is simply a temporary survival tactic. It's not something you should have to be doing all of the time over a long period of time.

How to effectively communicate your boundaries

Here are some strategies to support you through this practice of asserting your voice and navigating work situations, toxic or not:

- Be clear on whose opinions matter at the outset. Remember, not everyone's opinion matters. Think critically about who those key players are – whether it's about the people who strategically make a difference in making your job easier and help your career trajectory, or those whose opinions you value and respect. They don't have to be mutually exclusive, but those are some criteria to use to decide ahead of time.
- Choose the spaces and opportunities where you want to project yourself and own those spaces. There may be certain contexts in which you choose to be more selective and careful, but at least that is an active choice you're making and you're asserting agency over this. But also be sure to have environments where you can choose to speak up, say things without overcensoring, overqualifying, and diminishing yourself.
- Read/listen/talk to models of healthy boundary-setting and assertiveness skills. This is especially important for people from socially marginalized backgrounds.

The underfunctioner

Sometimes, becoming so preoccupied with what needs to be done at work can lead to shutting down and avoiding the endless amount of work. Chronic procrastination and other underfunctioning behaviors are incredibly common presentations of perfectionism at work. Take my client Peter's experience, for example.

Peter's manager gave him a set of tasks at the start of the week. He had a vague idea of when things should be done but looking at his list, he couldn't help but think, "Geez, this is . . . a lot." The ambiguity of timelines, tasks, and to whom he was accountable made it impossible to know what next steps he should take that day. He took a peek at his email inbox but again was left thinking, "Ugh, so many messages. I'll get to those later."

Would organizing his desk help him feel prepared to work? He got up, looked at his phone to check something online and then . . .

"And then hours passed and I hadn't made any progress on a single thing!" he sighed.

"What did you do in the meantime?" I asked.

"I responded to a few messages from coworkers on Slack. I kept hearing the ping of new email messages entering my inbox. More people added requests and meetings to my schedule. Whenever I had a thought that I should get started, my attention went to something else I could be doing. It never felt like the right time."

Peter described feeling angry at himself for not having made any progress and like he had "wasted the day." He told himself he'd try again the next day. But a part of him recognized, "I always do this. It's always the same."

If you recognized yourself in any parts of this scenario, please let me remind you this is not the time to judge yourself and criticize yourself for having done or thought any of these things. This is an amalgamation of so many people's experiences with getting stuck at work by the never-ending daunting list of responsibilities. You are not alone. Often people who view themselves as chronic procrastinators and "underperformers" ask me, "How did I get like this? How do I fix it? How do I just find more motivation?"

Some of the reasons this happens are because:

- unrealistic expectations fuel your need to get things done and simultaneously are the cause of you not doing much at all
- a lack of clear guidance and direction makes it hard for you to take concrete action
- you have a history of getting by in school or other jobs through a series of short-term, patch-work fixes – you don't address the root of the issue that drives your avoidance in the first place so you don't have the foundational skills to approach work differently
- there is a lot of shame built up around your past attempts at failing to "fix" your approaches to work and performance at work. Shame often leads to you isolating yourself and not asking for support.

Procrastination and seemingly "not doing anything" are in fact a reflection of the amount of pressure you put on yourself to get *so many things* done and done really well. Sometimes, in an attempt to rise to the occasion of "getting it all done" and perfect your performance, you will shut down and avoid work altogether because it all feels like too much. And that's not entirely wrong – it *is* too much!

What do you do with the feelings of overwhelm that lead to this procrastination cycle and spiral of avoidance?

The power of clarity

Clarity and specificity can help you avoid falling into per-fectionistic tendencies such as trying to reach the impossible goal of the "perfect" end state. Perfectionistic standards make it hard to know when something is "good enough" and the desire to do things "perfectly" will prevent you from getting started or knowing when to stop. I often hear people define their goal end state to "feel good enough" or "I want it to be just right." These are such non-specific outcomes – it's hard to quantify when you've reached a goal that's attached to a feeling. This is why it can often feel less than satisfying whenever you're trying to accomplish a task. Nothing feels *quite good enough yet*. There always seems to be a "yet" attached because more can always be done to improve it.

Strategies for managing expectations

- Be clear on what your expectations are and who has set them (are they external versus internal expectations?).
- Differentiate between the *actual* deliverables and timelines you're expected to abide by versus the *imagined* perfectionistic-driven outcomes and timelines you've created. The clearer you are on what is realistic, the better you can manage them appropriately.
- Double-check your projected task list and deadlines with someone else. Getting an outside perspective is useful in keeping expectations in check as well as giving you a source of support and accountability.
- Create a system for *how* you will get things done. It's common to get stuck when you look at your to-do list and think, "Where do I begin?" or "What is the next thing I'm supposed to do?" Ask yourself, "What is the immediate next thing I need to do to make the next step go smoother?" You're creating a domino effect by taking the first tiny action, then working closer to the next step, and so on.
- Be sure to document these steps – don't keep them in your head! Follow the documented steps like an instruction manual to guide you through your to-do list.

Strategies for reaching your goals

- Before you start a task, decide what will count as "done." This can be you deciding what done looks like for a single day's or hour's worth of work, not even the entire project.
- Write out detailed instructions and descriptions of what done looks like. This will help you know when to stop and what is "good enough."
- Have specific metrics and timelines to aim for. The more specific you get about what you want to have accomplished in what time frame, the better. If you tend to overdo tasks and don't usually have an issue with designating timelines and metrics, focus on scaling *down* the number and scaling *up* the timelines to make it more realistic. If you tend to underfunction and procrastinate, use specific metrics and realistic timelines to make the task approachable and the steps concrete.
- After looking at your list of tasks, go over it again with these questions to see where delegating, outsourcing, or delaying can be used:
  - Delegating: who else can do this with me or instead of me?
  - Outsourcing: what tool or system can I use that will make this task easier or irrelevant?
  - Delaying: does this need to be done within the next day or so or can I take this off my list so it's not a distraction from the priority items on my list?
- Find people with whom you can discuss your project time-lines and goals. These people can serve as sounding boards to double-check the realistic nature of your goals. They may also be able to offer alternative solutions and ways to get things done – perhaps they'll think of someone else who could take on one of your tasks, or a tool that will expedite

your work process. Asking for feedback from other people can be helpful. Others can see your to-do list from a perspective that's not imbued with a perfectionistic lens and they can offer solutions you may have trouble seeing or hadn't thought of.

Leila had a presentation due by Friday and it was Monday. She used the strategy of being specific with her "Done" list for the day and being clear on her expectations for today's task. She wrote to herself: Monday's Done = Create bullet points that will go on five presentation slides by 4 p.m.

She set a clear expectation to herself that today's slides would be rough drafts. This meant the bullet points could simply be "stream of consciousness" versions of the content that would eventually be captured on the presentation slides. She reminded herself, "Today is not about getting the content right. It is about getting content out."

She was clear on what her immediate next step would be. She wrote these words on a sticky note in plain sight: Step 1: Open a new presentation document and create five blank slides.

See how specific the details of the tasks were? And how clear her expectations were for herself? The next action step was small, doable and written down. The temptation may be to say, "That doesn't count" or "That's not enough." You need to temper that perfectionistic voice: "This is what I am choosing to be considered to be 'Done.'" This "talking back" to the perfectionistic voice is an active practice. Initially it may feel unnatural, but it's helpful to build up that muscle of asserting internal boundaries to how much work you're willing to put in at any given moment. You have to let these small, incremental actions count, otherwise you'll always be chasing something more. That is how we get to that place of overwhelm and start procrastinating or become burned out from overdoing.

The imposter

"Now I feel more pressure to prove myself and show that I deserve this promotion. I'm only as safe as how well I perform my job and avoid making any mistakes," my client shared the day after getting a promotion.

Instead of celebrating this milestone and feeling proud, she felt more anxious. As she continued to climb up the corporate ladder, she felt the stakes were getting higher. She felt even more vulnerable to getting found out as an imposter, someone who shouldn't be there. Midway through our session, she confessed, "Most times, I feel like I'm just one day away from getting fired."

Imposter syndrome is the feeling of achieving the role you're in because of a fluke, mistake, or pure luck. Imposter syndrome is a popular buzz term that describes so many people's experiences of not enoughness. Perfectionism and imposter syndrome are often brought up in tandem, especially pertaining to people's experiences in the workplace. People who are the most high-achieving, competent, and conscientious tend to fall into the trap of experiencing imposter syndrome.

I heard this from many students attending elite private institutions who felt they'd gotten in by mistake. I've heard this from successful women in leadership positions who fear it's only a matter of time until they're booted from their spots. Imposter syndrome makes it difficult to accept the strengths you have to offer because you're so bogged down by negative perceptions of yourself.

Research shows that people who experience imposter syndrome struggle to perform, not because they're less competent but because of the emotional and psychological toll it takes to navigate their work with this fear lingering over them. People from marginalized backgrounds always have this voice playing in the background: "Do I belong? Am I only here because I'm a minority hire?" That kind of mental toll is damaging and we see evidence of this in the numbers of people who remain stuck in the pipeline of academia and don't make it out on the other side. Most people who experience imposter syndrome are from marginalized communities. Often they don't come across models of successful people in positions of power so they aren't comfortable occupying those higher positions themselves. They don't feel as though they belong. And they're not entirely wrong in the sense that the systems put in place in education and many career institutions/industries often don't hire people of color or people with disabilities or other marginalized identities. So, it makes sense that someone would feel they don't belong because often they didn't in the past. There's a lot of history of segregation, exclusion, and other gatekeeping methods to prevent certain types of people from being hired, admitted into, and promoted to higher roles.

Imposter syndrome is a syndrome of systemic racism, sexism, ableism, and classism. Instead of internalizing a personal responsibility narrative that we're told – that it's our fault we're not succeeding or it's solely our responsibility to succeed and make it – it's important to consider the very real systemic responsibility or "fault" at play. There's a larger context you're embedded in that explains why you're feeling the way you do.

I acknowledge that simply having this systems-level view may not be enough to change your day-to-day situation. That being said, here are strategies to help you manage yourself within these inherently flawed systems.

How to manage imposter syndrome at work

1 Surround yourself with role models and supportive people. You need to have people around you who can validate, normalize, and strategize with you when things are hard. People who can also support you when you face incidents such as microaggressions or unjust work practices, or when it just straight up feels hard to exist at your job.

2 Find allies and positive connections who can encourage you and hold up a mirror of your value for you. Sometimes you need reminders from multiple sources.

3 Practice counter-beliefs to check the facts and do some "reality testing" of your competence. There's a difference between your degree of confidence versus your degree of competence. Usually with imposter syndrome, people are falsely putting too much weight on the belief that they're not competent when really they're just lacking confidence.

4 Practice self-affirming messages to yourself. Imposter syndrome rears its head through negative self-doubt thoughts. The imposter syndrome "voice" can get really loud. Counteract those messages of self-doubt with encouragement and reassurance. Here are some helpful reminders and messages to get you started:
   - Remind yourself how you got to where you are, how you deserve to be there, and what you have to gain and contribute by standing your ground in this position.
   - You have so much to offer by being someone in your role.
   - Don't waste your time worrying about whether or not you should be there. You're there now and it's time to do really great things.

5 Practice advocating for yourself. Take credit for what it is you're doing and make sure other people know too. Too

often, imposter syndrome leads to people diminishing their accomplishments. If you're convinced you shouldn't be there in the first place, you're less likely to consider you deserve more. Neither of those things is true, so it's important to work against those thoughts and do the opposite. Remind yourself you do deserve to be there *and* advocate for more.

In order to get ahead of the fear associated with the negative belief that you are "always on the brink of being found out," you might fall into, yet again, "hustling for your worth." This looks like you're constantly trying to prove your worth to yourself and to others through your job. You have a strong need for external validation, affirmation, and recognition to feel good enough. This happens when a perfectionist is not able to internalize and believe that they are good enough, but the above strategies should help you change your thinking.

The workaholic

"I wish I felt the kind of satisfaction I get from work in other areas of my life, but it's like a drug – nothing satisfies me like getting that positive feedback from the higher-ups at work, or when I get to walk into a room of impressive people and know I'm part of the 'club.'"

Despite the promotions to impressive C-suite title jobs, the higher salary, and getting access to privileges he knew were reserved only for those deemed "worthy" in his company, inside, Bruno didn't feel good enough.

Bruno's inner struggles to feel like he belonged or that he was good enough led him to become dependent on the external sources of validation he received from his job. He kept striving to occupy those high places and get rewarded for things at work in hopes of filling the void of inner enoughness.

This sense of "not enoughness" which we've discussed already gets tested a lot at work. People strive to feel like they're enough in the domain of their careers. I often hear my clients express how disappointed they feel when they fail to meet some standard at work. They tie so much of their worth and self-esteem to how they do at their job. They say things like:

- "If only I get that raise . . ."
- "If only I finish one more task . . ."
- "Just one more project – once this is off my plate, then I'll take some time off."

When you start to conflate performance and outcomes in your job with your internal sense of goodness, things get really dicey.

An addiction to external rewards and validation

Folks ride the "if only" train of thought over and over again when it comes to how they set expectations of themselves at work as well as what they expect to get done before they can "get back to their real life." This train doesn't tend to get people places other than a mental and physical state of burnout, disillusionment, and isolation. It is not to say that we shouldn't strive to accomplish certain things and set goals. But if it's perpetually used as a reason to delay living your life in a more fulfilling manner, or if it's used as a way to keep you overworking, then it's not helpful.

Bruno and I worked on disentangling his internal feelings and identity from the external "shiny" parts of the job and the external rewards he was getting from work. I helped him see that while his circumstances (being "let in" to inner circles) were positive benefits gained through his hard work and luck, those things were ultimately fleeting and outside of himself. He needed to focus more on the parts that were integral to who he was as a person and who he needed to pay attention to in order to live the other parts of his life in a present and whole-hearted way. Sure, he could enjoy the perks – nothing wrong with that – but he should not get caught up in thinking that was all he was worth or that he needed to keep striving to maintain that status and reach further. Because there's always more, further, shinier things . . .

In addition to the need to feel "good enough," other internal needs that fuel workaholism include:

- proving you are "good" and "worthy" by adding value and showing how you are good at things – as one client once put it, it's the need to prove that she was "worth her keep"
- needing to be needed (being seen as the go-to person at work)
- relying on the positive feelings you experience when you're told you are excelling and are deemed the high performer or star
- avoiding the harsh reality that you don't know what else you are good at outside of the skills you perform on the job, or who you are outside of your job title
- becoming accustomed to the "shiny" things or symbols of the "perfect" life. People talk about the "golden handcuffs," when the benefits (such as pay, promotions, status) get to be so tempting and harder to walk away from.

Now that we've discussed some of the common profiles of perfectionism at work, we will discuss some negative consequences of having unhealthy relationships to work and some issues that exacerbate these unhealthy relationships.

The loss of identity: "Who am I outside of work?"

You may fall into the group of people who have trouble separating their sense of worth from their job. Work makes up an outsized portion of their identity. Not only does it seem as though your identity is consumed by your job role or performance, this is also apparent through the way you schedule your time and experience your daily life. From the way you plan your days to who you spend the majority of your time interacting with, work is all-consuming.

Your self-worth/identity is not and cannot be wrapped up in your job, no matter how "passionate" you are. Be clear with yourself about the division between you and the work. You are not your work (regardless of whether this is work for someone else or yourself, whether it's a "passion" or not). You are not the sum of the output or achievements in your life. That's different and completely separate from you as a person. It can be an extension of your efforts and practice, but not an extension of who you are and your worth. This is a toxic message we get a lot from a system/society that needs us to think that our worthiness is equal to our output. Again, it's feeding the machine of capitalism and other powers, through our input.

Another message that's equally as problematic is that being productive is always a good thing, and falling short of that is somehow a negative reflection of our work ethic, discipline, or worthiness. There seems to be a cultural obsession with hyperproductivity and it keeps getting conflated with being a better person.

Examining your relationship to productivity

One of the reasons people struggle with investing in areas outside of work is because they think it's a waste of time. Our culture conditions us to think certain things are "productive" and "worthwhile" and others are a "waste." Leisure, hobbies, personal care, and social relationships get pushed aside while academic, professional development, work relationships, and job duties get put to the forefront of one's life. Just as I mentioned that my early work memories taught me what it means to be "productive," there are lots of cultural messages about productivity, hustling, and what are deemed as "good" uses of time.

Perfectionists spend a lot of time delivering in domains that receive approval. For most, that includes academic and professional settings. Activities that are deemed "good" are usually the ones that add to your career while the ones that are "just for fun" are frowned upon. This leads to people devaluing personal interests. When work and career-related activities become elevated, it makes sense that certain people's identities and whole lives get consumed by their jobs.

Reflection questions about your relationship to productivity

1 What is your relationship to time? For example, when do you tend to feel a scarcity of time versus an abundance of time?
2 What messages do you hold about "productivity"?
3 How do you rate your ability to "get things done"?
4 Looking back on your time at home and at school, which activities typically got approved and which were criticized?

You can practice mindfulness as you explore your overall narrative about work. Start by investigating the messages you internalized about what is considered "productive." Time management is more a matter of *attention* management. Therefore, it's important to know where your attention is going. Feel free to add your reflections on these prompts to your notes about your early work memories.

Doing the inner work of reclaiming your identity outside of work

Perfectionism is a form of trying to outperform feelings of low self-worth and constant self-doubt. Work is one domain of life where you can try to avoid feelings of not-enoughness. Rather than falling into the trap of proving your worth through work, you have to start with something hard but essential: *you have to do the inner work of addressing those self-doubts and insecurities that make you feel as though you have to prove yourself through work.*

This will help prevent you from falling back into the cycle of trying to "outperform" shame and low self-worth. Here are some strategies and reminders to help you build up a stronger internal sense of self and to mitigate the temptation to give more of yourself to work as a form of coping with those insecurities.

- Reduce your exposure to harmful messages that lead to more doubt and perfectionistic thinking patterns.
  - Be mindful of the messages you're exposed to about what is valuable and "worthy." If you constantly absorb cultural and societal messages saying you need to grind and overfunction to be successful, you're going to have a hard time *not* giving your life over to work. If you're only surrounded by people who can't set boundaries between their work and their personal life, you're going to be tempted to do the same. Divest from the "hustle and grind" culture!
  - Challenge your thought patterns about work/productivity and self-worth. Read and listen to other voices

that elevate other forms of well-being outside of doing more and "hustling." "Talk back to" that part of you that's still tempted to believe the more you do, the harder you work, the better you are. Instead, embrace messages that promote meaningful and reasonable expectations and taking care of your well-being outside of work.

- Focus on doing what you can that is manageable.
  - Put systems in place that will help you distinguish the time and attention boundaries between work and non-work responsibilities.
  - Regularly take stock of what you have done. Build in breaks between projects, rest periods in your day, and vacations to allow for space from work.
  - Don't be afraid to reach out for support and take advantage of tools that make doing the work easier.
- Be mindful of how you're associating work with your identity.
  - Instead of "If I complete x # of tasks, then I will feel better," remember that there will never be enough completed tasks to bring you a true sense of worthiness. Self-worth and acceptance do not come from the metrics of accomplishment. In the short term you'll feel that dopamine hit of satisfaction. But that's not the same thing as a long-lasting, grounded sense of well-being.
  - The next time you feel the temptation to give more of your precious resources to work, ask yourself: *What is it that I need to feel more grounded and confident in myself?*
  - Consider other sources of real well-being and invest your time and energy into those. Practice the things

that can soothe those feelings of stress, insecurity, and doubt. For example, if you've had a particularly stressful day, rather than just trying to muscle your way through more work-related tasks late into the night, consider eating a good meal, reading a book, and getting some needed sleep.

The fallacy of "work–life balance"

I often hear people state their desire to achieve "work–life balance." However, balance between the two domains of work and your personal life doesn't really exist. There's always going to be a tradeoff. Instead, the term "work–life balance" is more an issue of attention management and priority-setting.

One of the reasons people struggle to set priorities and manage their attention properly is because they're unwilling to let go of things at work. I believe this stems from a need to be in control of things and a sort of work FOMO. Work FOMO may not even really be about missing out but more a perception of *losing out* on certain opportunities. However, by trying to do so much and drowning as a result, you're actually working against your attempt to get ahead, gain opportunities. You have to be willing to let things go.

A strategy to help you not overdo and allow work to take over your life is to have clarity about your values. Your values influence the types of career goals you will set, specific job-related performance expectations, even down to how you'll go about interacting with people at your workplace. Values serve as guideposts to prevent you from straying too far from doing things in ways that serve you.

The harm in believing in "work as family"

One of the other reasons this melding of work and personal life can happen is when we buy into the "work as family," "work is my passion" narrative.

> "I don't want to let people down at work," one client told me. "They've become like family to me. If I don't handle these issues at work, then I feel bad because it's going to fall onto my colleagues. I respect them and I don't want to make their lives harder. I can just handle these things myself."

These types of statements are often what my clients say to me when they're struggling to let go of responsibilities that either don't belong to them or they feel are too much on their plate. It's a common misconception that just because you get along with your coworkers, you respect and like your boss, then you need to be even more accommodating to them. It's not a matter of being liked or liking other people. It's a matter of separating your work and all of the components of your work, including the relationships in them, from what you choose to do in your broader life. You have to be able to separate what needs to be done to take care of yourself and the people in your non-work life versus what needs to be done within the confines of your job.

Perfectionism and people-pleasing can intersect to make people overfunction and over-accommodate at work. The relationships at work become another reason that people start to do more than they need to and should. People want to please everyone but especially the people they like and deem to be "friends" and maybe "like family."

I balk at terms referring to people at work as family, "work wives," or similar tropes. While it's sort of cute to think of the people you spend so much time with in endearing terms, it's not actually helpful. In fact, it's harmful. Because think about the kinds of things you're willing to do for your actual friends and family. You're most likely willing to go above and beyond and make sacrifices for them because you care a lot about them, right? But what happens when you start to attribute this term "family" to people at work? Soon you're making sacrifices for pretty much everyone in your life. It starts to muddy the waters of who earns the right of family and those accommodations you make for them. It muddies the boundaries between *actual* family versus non-family.

Stop referring to people at work as "family" or anything in that vein. Language matters and how you think and refer to people will translate into the ways you decide to engage with them. The language you use to refer to people in your life can contextualize the place they fit into in your life. So, for example, your boss will never be your "work dad" or something similar. Your boss will remain "the boss." You have a mental model for what a relationship between you and your boss looks like. A boss gets the hours of your day that are agreed upon (let's say, 9 a.m. to 5 p.m.) and nothing more than that, with rare exceptions. Your boss should not get those outside-of-work hours that are dedicated to yourself and your community (e.g. friends, family, others).

Similarly, a coworker may be a "work friend" or "work colleague" but not a "wifey" or something like that. This can impact the way you engage with them both during work and after. How much you disclose with them about your personal life is up to you, but you will most likely make certain decisions that differentiate them from your actual friends outside of work.

The role of toxic work culture in driving perfectionism

Perfectionists can be easy targets of toxic work culture because of overdoing, overfunctioning, and people-pleasing. Perfectionists can overlook the flags of toxic work culture and relationships and have an increased risk of minimizing their boundaries.

Some flags to recognize in work culture include:

- a lack of transparency
- constantly moving targets
- inequitable treatment of and benefits for workers
- expectation of overwork and self-sacrifice
- harsh and critical interactions among coworkers and managers
- lack of respect for people's schedules (during and after work).

Some red flags to recognize in colleagues include:

- perfectionistic bosses and coworkers
- micro-managers
- volatile and unpredictable people
- emotionally manipulative people who abuse power to get others to do things.

Unfortunately, when we're so set on trying to meet people's expectations and be seen as good, hardworking, compliant, high-performing individuals, we can miss those warning signs of boundary-crossing, disrespectful, and unjust work behavior and conditions.

However, it's not just the inability to see the signs. Sometimes even if you see something is wrong and identify problems, you are at a loss as to how to get out of the situation. This is where remembering that larger socio-cultural forces outside of our individual selves are often complicit in making these problematic situations possible. Being in toxic situations is not your fault. However, as I mentioned before and I repeatedly remind my clients, it is your responsibility to find ways to get out.

Perfectionists need to see things more clearly for what they are, not what they could be if they only worked harder or were responsible for fixing them. Some things are *not* about you outperforming certain conditions. Overcoming the fear of failure and conflict allows you to take more risks and assert yourself more clearly. This shift in mindset will translate into how you live your life, such as how you manage your schedule, what commitments you hold, and where your resources go. Example phrase: "I commit to only giving *this* much, no more and no less."

How to navigate toxic work situations

- Work with allies and build a community (in-person and virtual) via affinity groups, coaching, mentorship.
- Practice self-advocacy skills.
- Get support outside of work in therapy and/or with friends who care about your well-being who can help you game plan ways to navigate or leave situations when need be.
- Remember, you can leave situations and find better opportunities (you are not stuck!).

Create rules of engagement

Creating and implementing rules of engagement is a form of exercising your autonomy and agency over the domain of work. "Rules of engagement" are a set of boundaries and expectations for yourself and others when it comes to work. The clearer your boundaries are and the more specific you can be about your rules, the better it will be for you and the relationships in your life. People who maintain healthy boundaries at work are often the most grounded and generous. They're able to do this because they can set themselves internal rules about what is and isn't okay. When they have clarity on that for themselves, they can do a better job of translating that out to the world via their actions and words.

1 What are some rules or guidelines for how you get things done as you are working?
2 What are some rules or guidelines you can set in place for how you approach relationships at work?
3 What are some rules or guidelines for how you manage your time and attention between work and personal life?

For inspiration, think about models of healthy relationships and boundaries you've seen other people practice in their professional lives. What stands out to you about those people? They may be people who can separate their personal self from their professional self by the way they talk about aspects of their lives – the degree to which they disclose things, how they're judicious about personal information, and how they're not fishing for it from other people. They may abide by strict out-of-office boundaries with their time and attention – they don't respond to emails outside of work hours and support others to do the same. They arrive and leave the office (virtual or in person) at consistent and reasonable times, and they allow for flexibility for personal issues that arise.

Suggested guidelines for engaging with work include:

- Be more mindful of how you think about and refer to your work colleagues and supervisors. Notice the language you've used to describe people. Practice being more deliberate about using language that matches the context. Repeat after me: You are not your job, nor is your workplace your "family."

- Agree to yourself the kind of information you'd like to share with colleagues. There may be some things you have no problem talking about pretty openly. Some topics you might prefer to keep to yourself with rare exceptions – when it'll make things easier and clearer if you were to share minimal information. Some topics will be strictly off limits and you will not discuss them at work.

How to change your approach to work

A "good enough" approach can help reclaim your life from the grips of perfectionism in work. I notice that for perfectionists who are high achievers and want to be the best, better, and great, the term "good enough" can be unsatisfying, bordering on insulting/sad – a kind of settling for being worse off. But I challenge people to consider what's so wrong with good enough. Even your definition of what good enough looks like can be another person's great. What matters is what it'll take for you to get to that place of good enoughness, not just at work but also internally.

If it requires you to sacrifice your health and well-being to achieve your standard of great, and you're not really living your life to get that brief satisfaction associated with "great," then is it that bad to go for good enough? It can be a relief from that constant striving and overtaxing of your body and mind when you present this alternative – that you can be good enough at your job *and* live a good, maybe even a great (!), life outside of your job. I'd love for you to make that tradeoff.

Reflection questions: re-evaluating our relationships with work

It's time to decide what sorts of messages about work you want to carry forward. Here are some questions to help you re-evaluate work in your life:

1 How do you want to feel when it comes to work?
2 How is it that you want to feel while you're at your job (whether it's this one or some other job in the future), with people you work with?
3 How do you want your job to fit into the overall picture of your life?
4 Based on how it looks now, is there something you want to change?

List the feelings, the vision of how you want your life to look, and any of the changes you thought of. Your responses can center on how you'd like to feel, how you'd like to schedule your life, how you would like your relationships both at work and in your personal life to look. This exercise may lead you to think about what you might be doing for work altogether. Perhaps you'll realize you don't like your job or industry and you can write down the possibility of a career pivot in the near future.

There are no wrong or right answers. For perfectionists who like concrete solutions and clear directions, exercises like these can be disorienting. "What do you mean I can say and think whatever I want?" Remember, these reflection questions are meant to be notes to yourself. Take a curious observer-like stance and don't judge what comes to mind.

The answers to these questions may illuminate some surprising things. I hope so. I know that whenever I re-evaluated my relationship with work, I experienced a range of emotions. My clients, too, have described these reflection exercises as scary, exciting, illuminating, surprising, not surprising, empowering, daunting, and refreshing.

Keep these notes handy. We'll return to them later in the book when we delve deeper into how values will guide the way we engage with aspects of our lives beyond the scope of work.

Having a good enough relationship with work

Remember Kai and how she was so sick of feeling like a pushover? She came to therapy feeling completely burned out and demoralized from years of overdoing at her job with little to show for it in her personal life. Our work together allowed her to decouple her identity from what she delivered at work, and from the status symbols she worked so hard to achieve. She learned that being proud of those accomplishments and the sacrifice she made to get there could co-exist with a life outside of these things.

We took time to rediscover other parts of herself. In order to be able to step away bit by bit from her job, she needed to have something to step away to. This meant doing the harder work of trying new things, reaching out and interacting with old friends, and building new friendships. She learned she actually preferred cooking rather than getting takeout delivered to her office every day. She learned she liked all things journals and stationery, so she picked up a hobby of handwriting journals and loved visiting stationery stores on the weekends. She began casually dating just to see what it would be like to meet people outside of work, experience the city she'd been living in all those years, and to talk about anything else besides work. The more she set boundaries with coworkers on her time and availability for job-related functions and tasks, the more she realized it was time to look for another job. There were some successes getting people to respect her boundaries, but the amount of pushback signaled to her that this wasn't a respectful and good-fit work environment for her anymore. She found another job, which also helped remind her that she had a lot to offer and she didn't need to remain stuck in unhealthy environments.

Building awareness of how and when perfectionism shows up in your relationship to work will help you get ahead of whatever old habits and patterns used to emerge. You can choose how to respond in ways that make more room for your identity outside of work. This can look like investing more attention into other areas of your life. You can let go of the belief "I am only as good as the output of my job." Next, we'll examine how perfectionism can also show up in our relationships, another domain of our lives where many perfectionists garner a sense of worth and identity.

4
Perfectionism in relationships

Introduction

When it comes to relationships, perfectionists can feel like they're in a bit of a bind. On the one hand, the traits that make them perfectionists – the high standards, conscientiousness, high functioning, and the tendency towards performing at their best for others – can be the exact things that make them the "ideal" relationship partner. People on the receiving end of a perfectionist's behaviors can feel taken care of and they may be attracted to these sacrificial, selfless behaviors. On the other hand, when done this way constantly, those overused perfectionistic tendencies can lead to the person feeling tired, used, and dissatisfied.

There needs to be a more realistic and balanced approach to relationships that a perfectionist can take. It shouldn't have to require becoming burned out or having to avoid relationships completely.

- "I don't know who I am outside of the things I can do for others."
- "It's weird. I have a lot of friends but I still feel so empty and like no one really gets me."
- "Isn't it normal to want to take care of everyone? I just care a lot. But I also don't feel like I can keep going at this rate."
- "Sometimes I think it would be easier if I didn't care so much about the people in my life. I feel horrible saying that, but I'm just so sick and tired of taking on everyone else's stuff. When do I get a break?"

In Chapter 3, we discussed how perfectionism leads to striving for external validation through work. Personal and professional relationships as a whole serve as a major source of external validation. This chapter will delve deeper into how perfectionism affects our approach to relationships. This discussion of relationships includes everything from early childhood relationships, dating relationships, and friendships to the professional and other encounters that fall somewhere in between.

Many perfectionists identify as "people-pleasers" and we'll talk about where people-pleasing tendencies come from. Various traits and tendencies emerge under the umbrella of people-pleasing within relationships, including:

- overfunctioning
- caretaking
- fear of boundaries and conflict
- fear of vulnerability
- not asking for help
- acting solely out of obligation, not from one's values.

When these relationship patterns persist, associated risks and negative outcomes include:

- burnout
- resentment
- feeling stuck
- remaining in unhealthy, toxic relationships
- lack of self-awareness.

Throughout the chapter I will weave in typical examples from people I've encountered who illustrate these relationship struggles rooted in perfectionism. As always, I'm coming at this topic from a cultural lens and I'll include examples of how intergenerational and cultural factors intersect with the expectations we internalize as well as what we believe is possible when it comes to things like setting boundaries, asserting ourselves, and speaking up for our needs.

There is a world in which you can maintain close relationships without having to burn yourself out or feel resentful. You can make intentional choices about how you show up in relationships. I'll include strategies and things to think about when it comes to overcoming old scripts about how we should engage in our relationships, as well as how to practice changing behaviors and navigating relationships differently. I want you to consider your needs as equal to those you care about and to practice making room for yourself in relationships. That being said, I'm aware of how most advice tends to come from a solely Eurocentric mentality, so I have included an array of options for responding to situations rather than a one-size-fits-all approach.

The umbrella people-pleaser

You can't throw a stone too far from perfectionism without hitting people-pleasing. A large part of how we see ourselves has to do with how we get along with other people. We figure out ways we need to behave in order to gain approval and to feel that people like us. Just as we've discussed how perfectionists strive to do things "right," a perfectionistic approach to relationships opens up another world of "should." Some relationship-specific shoulds include:

- I should be someone who gives freely and generously to others.
- I should be someone who will say yes to requests because that's the nice thing to do.
- I should be someone who is accommodating to the needs of other people.
- I should be someone who avoids conflict and disagreements; these are "bad" situations.

- I should be someone who avoids speaking up or asking for what I need if it could cause more trouble for others.
- I should be someone who takes care of myself; being independent is far better than being "needy" and "weak."

You may try to abide by this series of unspoken and spoken relationship shoulds based on the unrealistic assumption that you need to adhere to them all of the time or else you're not doing relationships "right." When you operate under that assumption without question, this can damage you and your relationships. No human being, no matter how caring and well-intentioned, can realistically "do relationships perfectly" all the time without at some point feeling somewhat weighed down and eventually downright resentful.

Perfectionism, as we will discuss in more depth in Chapter 6, has its benefits. I often hear people describe themselves as empathic, sensitive, and caring, as perfectionists will go to great lengths to make people around them feel good. However, the drawbacks appear when perfectionists devote themselves completely to every relationship regardless of its quality.

Instead, we need to stop and examine where we adopted these rules. When we better understand the root of our patterns of behavior in relationships, we can choose differently and make intentional choices about how we engage in our relationships. So, where did your relationship shoulds come from?

Early relationship memories

Just as we dug into some early work-related memories, I want you to do the same with relationships.

1 How do you define what being "good" in a relationship looks like? How do you define being a good partner, child, parent, colleague, and/or friend?

2 What are your earliest positive memories of relationships? What stood out to you and what did you learn from these people and interactions?

3 What are your earliest negative memories of relationships? What stood out to you and what did you learn from these people and interactions?

4 Name some significant relationship role models who taught you what it means to be "good" in relationships. If nothing personal comes to mind, you can include things you learned through media and stories.

How our families serve as the earliest models of relationships

Many of my clients describe their early childhood experiences as pivotal learning grounds for their relationship patterns. We take away a lot from what we observe in the parental figures, elders, and other close adult caregivers we were surrounded by. As you reflected on your early relationship memories that taught you what a "good" or "unhealthy"/"bad" relationship was, how many of you wrote that some sort of family member was a significant influence in your life?

This exercise of reflecting on the past can help you recognize patterns you adopted from people and early experiences that maybe you weren't fully aware of. It's also nice to remember the positive influences in our lives that led to us being who we are today.

Next, let's consider your present-day relationship patterns.

Your current relationship patterns

1 When it comes to being in relationships, what are your strengths?

2 What do you struggle with when it comes to relationships?

3 How do you think your early relationships and the lessons you took away from those may be tied to your current strengths and weaknesses in your relationships?

Use these questions to explore the past and how it connects to your present-day relationship patterns. This exploration process will eventually allow you to make intentional choices about what is worth carrying forward and what's better to let go.

Next, we will delve into some common profiles of individuals struggling with perfectionistic approaches towards and beliefs about their relationships.

Relationship archetypes for perfectionists

Archetype	Definition
The "Hyper-independent"	*I can do it myself, I don't rely on others.*
The "Strong One"	*Asking for help is too risky. I don't want people to see me as weak. I don't like to open up because then they won't like me.*
The "Caretaker"	*My value is only as good as my ability to take care of everyone else and make their lives better and easier.*
The "Martyr"	*I do so much for other people and what do I get in return? No one else is going to do it, so I have no choice but to do it myself.*

The hyper-independent type

"I've learned not to rely on other people for anything. I don't have to deal with the disappointment of people not being able to give me what I want or making me feel bad because I asked for something."

Growing up, her mom often used my client's requests against her. Her mother would make it about the burden her daughter placed on her. She refused to listen to my client. She refused to meet her needs.

Because this interaction kept happening over and over again, my client eventually figured it was better to just take care of everything herself.

In her session with me, she finished, "I just don't want to feel like I owe anyone anything."

Some perfectionists go at everything alone because they learn it's "better this way." In the case of my client whose words you see above, her hyper-independent nature stemmed from her childhood experiences. It made sense that over time, my client developed an aversion to the idea of asking for her needs and expressing herself.

This kind of reaction and adaptive coping strategy is common in these types of problematic relationship experiences. In the short term, it's a good solution to avoid unpleasant situations. But in the long term, it can become damaging because it forgoes your needs. My client's adaptive coping mechanism was ultimately at her own expense when it led to her stopping advocating for herself or sharing much of herself with others.

For my client, another unfortunate consequence of this early experience with her mom was that my client internalized that *she* was the problem and therefore fixing *her* behaviors would be the solution. I consider this unfortunate because it wasn't true that my client was the problem. The real culprit was her mom's lack of emotional maturity and inability to make space for anyone other than herself. Some people don't have the emotional maturity and capability to listen to someone else's needs and opinions without making it about themselves. This stems from a scarcity mindset and the limiting belief that having to fulfill someone else's needs, even if it's just to listen to them, will somehow make their lives harder.

It's not your fault

Recognizing that you're embedded in this dynamic with someone who lacks the skills to engage in a shared relationship with you is half the battle. Now, you can start to differentiate the parts of the scenario that have nothing to do with you. Even though you may have been made to feel like asking for something or speaking up was a "problem," you can start to see the situation through a different lens. The point is not to assign blame but to distance yourself from taking on full responsibility for a situation that's not yours to hold. When you no longer believe old messages that you were "bad" for having shared or asked for something, you can consider trying those behaviors again with more self-compassion.

It can be an emotional process to start recognizing that it was someone else's shortcomings that were responsible for some problematic tendencies. On the one hand, it can feel liberating. Many of my clients have expressed hope and relief that they were not as bad as they were made to feel. On the other hand, I've heard feelings of sadness, anger, and guilt in response to this process of introspection. The sadness and anger can be reactions to an unfair situation that played out for a long time, maybe decades. The guilt can arise when the people we're talking about in these dynamics are people we care about deeply or towards whom we feel a sense of loyalty. It's not always easy to see some emotional shortcomings in others. But identifying what is yours versus someone else's is essential in reclaiming your rightful place in relationships.

The strong one

Similar to hyper-independent types, some perfectionists fear that asking for help or sharing emotionally vulnerable parts of themselves will make people think they are weak. They strive to appear "strong" and "put together." But this is based on appearances, not reality. Part of being authentic in your relationships means you need to be willing to show up as you are, including when you feel less than your best. This includes times you're in need, you're struggling, you've made a mistake, or you're unsure of what to do. Perfectionism creates this narrative that all of those things are horrible and should be hidden from plain sight. However, this is so far from what is true of our human experience. We're all flawed and a bit confused at times, and that's okay. We need to make room for that in ourselves and for each other.

When you put on this front that you're doing all of the "right things" and "have it all together" on the inside, that strong facade can actually make you seem closed off or unapproachable. Many of my clients struggle with fears of being vulnerable. They feel unfulfilled and misunderstood by others. I also hear from people who are on the receiving end of someone else behaving that way. For both parties, the result is the same: people experience the relationship as shallow and can feel an emotional distance between themselves and the other person.

The fear of vulnerability is based on myths that showing emotions, expressing needs, and sharing challenges one is experiencing is "weak" or "needy." These are undesirable traits to someone who strives to be seen as perfect, strong, and put together. Instead, sharing and mutuality in relationships are cornerstones to building intimacy and closeness. People understand one another better if they know more than just surface-level information. Vulnerability leads to stronger connections and it takes a lot of courage. Societal biases about what is deemed "strong" are paired with masculine traits and being "weak" with feminine traits. It's important to question these assumptions and biases that limit how we express ourselves and to accept a full range of emotions and human experiences.

When we're able to accept our strengths' and weaknesses and disentangle them from any notion of perfection, we can more readily let others see those parts of us too. This gives way to building deeper relationships based on acceptance and respect, not shallower relationships based on surface-level appearances and performative behaviors of what seems "good" (i.e. perfect).

Practice being vulnerable by opening up and being more honest about what's on your mind. This doesn't mean you have to perpetually "fall apart" in front of everyone all of the time. There's a difference between dumping on someone because you can't regulate your emotions versus deliberately choosing to share something about yourself with someone. There are more appropriate times, places, and people for being vulnerable. Remember, being a good relationship partner means you can be honest about your needs, accept the fact that you make mistakes and struggle at times. It takes all parties being present and engaged to succeed. That includes you, "warts and all!"

The caretaker

"I didn't have a choice but to figure out how to take care of myself and my brothers," my client told me. "My mom didn't have the capacity to do more. She was working two jobs; I never saw her. Even if I needed something, who would hear it?"

Raised by a single mother, my client was put in this caretaking role from a young age. She had two siblings and was both explicitly and implicitly told that she had to take care of them.

"I'm only as good as my service to other people," she continued. She was known among friends and family as the go-to person. She said yes to everyone's requests and often took on the bulk of the responsibilities.

I gently asked, "Why don't you let other people help you?"

She shook her head, saying, "It's just easier if I do it myself. Or usually, it's something that only I can do."

Due to her early childhood experiences, my client became someone whose identity was wrapped up in being a caretaker for everyone in her life. As an adult, she struggled to see herself outside of being useful to people, and she always had an excuse for why no one else but her could be the caretaker.

My client felt lost without fulfilling the duties and responsibilities from which she garnered a sense of self-worth and value. It was painful to recognize that without being useful to others, she felt people wouldn't accept her or want her to be a part of their lives.

Reclaiming your personal identity

This loss of a personal identity is a very real risk for people-pleasers. Because their identity has been so tied to what they can do for other people, people-pleasers have to rediscover who they are outside of what they provide for others.

Rediscovering who you are and building up your personal identity is a process. It is a process of getting to know yourself not unlike getting to know a new friend. What do you do when you meet someone new? You ask questions, you get curious about what they enjoy, what lights them up, what they value, and how they like to spend their time and energy.

May I remind you that so many people are going through this process, sometimes at multiple points throughout their lives, and therefore you don't have to feel alone. Getting to know yourself can be both nerve-wracking and exciting. It is helpful to do this in a guided manner, either through writing if you're a journaler, or with someone else if you like to process things out loud. Therapy, close friendships, or coaches can all serve as helpful sounding boards for when you're rediscovering parts of yourself.

Once you know yourself better and identify who you are outside of your relationships, you can identify things you need and want. But what happens when you feel you don't deserve to have those needs met? How does one go from doing so much for others to giving themselves permission to ask for more? Here we can see how the scarcity mindset and perfectionism intersect with our relationships.

Perfectionism as a form of scarcity in relationships

The sense of scarcity and not feeling deserving of more is something perfectionists have to overcome in many domains of their lives, including relationships. Perfectionism can make you feel you don't have a right to ask for what you want. This can be because you've come to believe you're lucky even to have whatever you have, or that you're not entitled to more since you have "enough" now. However, you can be fortunate, have enough, *and* still make requests for things in your life. This can be hard to believe because, again, we've been told by others that this isn't true.

How culture and society contribute to the scarcity mindset

"You shouldn't make trouble for other people."

"You're a child, so you don't have a say in this matter. Other people know more than you, including things about yourself."

There are messages such as the ones above that make perfectionists and people-pleasers feel they deserve only a limited amount of attention or space. People in positions of authority commonly add, "This is what's best for you." While this may be rooted in good intentions, it can quickly become harmful when it is overused across all situations. Soon it becomes less a sentiment rooted in what is actually "best" and more a way to dismiss and silence you.

These silencing and dismissing tactics used by other people, intended or not, can underlie your inability to trust your feelings and opinions. Perfectionists try to do their best in all situations, particularly in relationships. You don't want to "rock the boat" or "stir up trouble." So, if you're told that staying silent, not asking for your needs, and settling for what you have is "best" for you and those around you, you'll be more apt to listen and take it in as truth.

Most people-pleasing is based on the assumption that it's a win-win for everyone if you just do what you're told and don't question things. You might assume, "If I just give them what they want, won't everything be fine?" But this is not necessarily the case. Maybe in the short term, but often in the long run, problems arise. This is because when you people-please, you're usually making an even deeper assumption that whoever is making the rules definitively knows what is "best" in a given situation. Perfectionists may not stop to question whether or not they have a valuable perspective to offer, or that speaking up and adding their opinions and feelings may be useful.

I want to pause and acknowledge that certain cultural and societal expectations play a large role in why we choose not to speak up and offer our perspectives. This is common in the general category of "collectivistic" cultures, such as the Asian cultural upbringing I had. I was not encouraged to chime in with my opinions and perspectives when it came to making decisions in our household. Even later, when I'd surpassed American markers of "adulthood," I still wasn't considered an adult in my family of origin. Not in a way that would merit my input at the same level as that of my parents or other adults in our community. There remained a separation between "the adults" and "the kids" among our family friends and relatives. If I wanted to remain in the "in-group," I couldn't risk offending people, which meant I shouldn't speak out of turn.

Stay small, "don't rock the boat"

My clients have shared similar sentiments about being told, "Don't rock the boat," "Don't make trouble," and "You only deserve this much. You're lucky to even have this much, so don't ask for more." As a result, they became completely averse to anything resembling conflict. They aimed to make themselves smaller, which meant not advocating for themselves and only taking the minimal amount of resources they could get by on, whether that was time, attention, or money. This is especially true for people from marginalized backgrounds, such as queer, Black, Indigenous, People of Color (BIPOC), and low-income folks. The sense of scarcity they're so used to experiencing in childhood or at home can often lead to the misconception that what little they have is all they deserve.

I recognize that remaining small in relationships can sometimes be a coping mechanism. Similar to other coping mechanisms we develop, it serves a helpful function in the short term, but such mechanisms are only good when they fit the situation. Sometimes the strategy of being small is no longer useful. How do you know when your coping strategy has expired? Let's turn to some negative consequences of staying small and operating from this scarcity mindset in relationships.

The slow build-up of resentment

The perfectionistic tendencies towards suppressing your needs, overfunctioning, and not asserting boundaries can only go so far until you and your relationships feel the negative consequences: resentment, burnout, misunderstandings, and conflict.

Resentment is a very real potential outcome for folks who overfunction and give so much of themselves to others in relationships. This is something you need to look out for in your relationships if you want to maintain connections over the long term. Resentment builds over time. It's easy to miss the rise of these feelings until it's too late. The way to prevent it from accumulating is by being mindful of the warning signs.

Warning signs of resentment include related emotions and reactions such as bitterness, irritability, and annoyance. I've heard people describe a looming sense of dread and "heaviness" similar to persistent tiredness and exhaustion beneath the surface as they go about their daily life. Think about the times you felt similar emotions. What do you think they were signaling to you about how you were operating in your life? What part of those feelings had to do with the relationship work you were doing?

The martyr

My client grew up with parents who fought constantly. She was an "emotional punching bag" for her mom and the "receptacle" of chaos in her family. During her mom and dad's many conflicts, they left duties at home, such as housekeeping, by the wayside. Reflecting on that time, my client told me tearfully, "It didn't matter what I wanted. I still had to get things done. If I didn't, who else would?"

As an adult, my client was overfunctioning. She was doing things for people in her life both at home and at work even though she did not want to do them. "If I don't do everything, everything will fall apart. I feel like it's me against the world and I'm all alone."

When I asked her why she didn't ask for help, she said everyone else was incapable. Her partner asked how he could chip in, but she refused to rely on him. She was someone who could "do it herself."

However, "doing it herself" was depleting her physical and emotional energy. The harder she pushed herself to get things done, the more her resentment built up. She struggled with constant feelings of disappointment from unmet expectations. "Why do I always have to fix other people's mistakes? Am I the only one who can get things done well around here?"

My client was falling into a spiral of victimization and a sense of isolation. Her tendency to take on things by herself came from her upbringing. From a young age, she internalized that she needed to shoulder the burden and pick up the slack because of other people's inability to take care of themselves or her. But she obviously did not enjoy those responsibilities. She seemed almost defeated when she admitted how painful the experiences were and how hard it was to grow up with those expectations. We named those expectations of herself she had long held and how she'd begun projecting them onto everyone else. Once she could recognize them, it became easier for her to see how those unrealistic expectations were setting up everyone else for failure and herself for feeling disappointed and resentful.

Perfectionists start to see their high, unrealistic metrics as "normal," especially when those standards go unchallenged and rewarded in society. They start to hold other people to those same metrics. But you and other people are not the same, with the same resources, values, or abilities. Therefore, holding others to the same unrealistic standards you hold yourself to isn't helpful and can easily lead to those dreaded feelings of disappointment and resentment. Being judgmental and critical is not something perfectionists consciously choose to do. Of course, no one *wants* to treat themselves or others this way! However, the stress of trying to do things perfectly can override our wiser empathic side and our ability to think big picture. It's easy to become so self-focused that you lose sight of seeing yourself and other people as fully human, with flaws and unique circumstances.

How to overcome a tendency towards martyrdom and prevent resentment

It takes conscious thought and practice to recalibrate your expectations of yourself and others. Be clear on your expectations and change them to become more realistic. This includes becoming more adaptable, less attached to outcomes, and scaling them appropriately.

Commit to doing things only when you're in the right mind, body, and emotional space. If you can agree to something, then go right on ahead. Pause before saying yes to a request and ask if you're having any of the following thoughts:

• I should.
• It's always been done this way.
• No one else will do it if I don't.
• I can do it better.

It is not a matter of whether or not any of these statements are true. Even so, none of those reasons is enough to keep up this habit of overdoing from a place of resentment and bitterness.

Adopt a me-first mentality. You can't give what you don't have. If you want to keep showing up for people in your relationships with a greater sense of well-being and appreciation, you need to take care of yourself first. Perfectionists often have a hard time accepting the me-first mentality because it goes counter to the things they were taught to believe. You may fear that taking up space in the relationship means you are taking away from someone else. In reality, by putting yourself first, you'll be able to generate more not only for yourself but for others. It is not a zero-sum game.

Let go of the scarcity mindset that says there is not enough time, space, emotional resources, love, etc. to go around. It takes some undoing of those old narratives to start practicing a more abundant and generous mindset/approach to relationships. There is enough room for both. Believing this and practicing this generous mindset requires trust – trusting that other people can share the relationship with you.

Reconnecting and reclaiming your self

A people-pleaser's relationship shoulds coupled with their desire to do things perfectly lead to using up their energy and time for others and losing sight of what their own needs are. Overdoing, becoming so consumed by the need to please and give to others, and feeling burned out or resentful, will quickly disconnect you from your body and mind. In order to reconnect to your needs, you must reclaim your time and energy. This is easier said than done, but it can happen in practical ways – including speaking up for yourself, setting boundaries, and making intentional choices about how you're spending your time. Before we talk about practical ways to reclaim your time, I want to add an important discussion about common advice about relationships.

The problem with generic advice: when it's not that simple

"I hear so much talk about 'setting boundaries' and how I 'should' be able to tell my parents off because I'm a so-called adult, but it's not that simple. I don't feel like this advice fits for me. It's more complicated than that."

I speak from personal life experience as well as from counseling others that a one-size-fits-all approach to setting boundaries or communicating needs isn't helpful. Statements such as "Just do what you want" or "You're an adult, therefore you don't have to adhere to those rules or perform obligations" don't make sense for everyone when there are cultural and generational messages to consider. This struggle comes up a lot with children of immigrant families and people of color who came of age in a generation and a culture that clash with those of their parents. This misfit between generic advice and people's circumstances is a result of advice given from predominately Eurocentric, heteronormative, and gender-stereotyped perspectives. Those perspectives hold certain assumptions about what people are capable of exercising in their lives.

Another problem with generic advice is how it's presented – in very black-and-white terms, and without much room for a process to unfold, a natural give and take. Instead, it's directive: "Do this, don't do that." You're left with the sense that if you don't do something immediately, you won't fix the problem right away. However, relationships are complicated, they're dynamic, and change takes time.

It can be very frustrating if you try to apply well-meaning but generic advice to your situation and feel as though things get worse. You may feel more hopeless about changing the original situation. This is why I am presenting a *culturally-informed perspective* to managing perfectionism, people-pleasing, and meeting expectations with a more nuanced approach to setting boundaries. I believe it is possible to maintain connections to your close relationships, honor your cultural values, and preserve your sense of well-being. It will take more creativity, flexibility, and patience to find what feels appropriate for you depending on the cultural background, traditions, and values you grew up with. A culturally-sensitive and realistic approach to finding boundaries that fit your relationships will take into account these multiple factors.

A culturally informed not "one-size-fits-all" approach to relationships

Here are some aspects to consider when figuring out how to set boundaries with people who may not be of the same generation and cultural upbringing or on the same page as you when it comes to your relationship.

1 Who is the "receiver" of the boundary?

You're going to approach your elderly grandmother differently than you do your younger sister. You're going to approach your romantic partner who grew up in the same social context as you differently than you will a colleague who is of a different racial background and is much older. It may seem obvious, but being clear on this at the outset will help you take the appropriate approach to a relationship conflict or conversation.

2 What is it that you want to see happen and what is it that you want to stop?

Be clear on what these two things are – it can be helpful to name both what you want more of and what you want less of. People respond better to being told what they *can* do as opposed to what they can't or shouldn't do. Give people a direction to move towards, like a more appropriate way to speak to you or a more useful way to help.

3 What are your expectations about the potential outcomes and consequences of making this request?

It's good to go in having thought about what your expectations are. Being realistic about how someone may respond and being able to plan ahead a bit can reduce the anxiety you might feel about approaching this person. Also, you can manage your expectations accordingly and have a contingency plan if things go differently or less ideally.

The impact of generational and cultural differences in our approach to relationships

My clients often say "this is just how they are" about their family members. Navigating differences in people's values and upbringings can be tricky. This is not something you can go in trying to change right away or maybe at all. There's a difference between asking someone to see a situation from your perspective, which they may not be willing or able to do, versus asking someone to act in a more appropriate way. Both can feel like a challenge, but one is more realistic than the other.

They also say, "I don't feel like I can handle this conversation right now." Sometimes it can just be too much or not the time to get into a discussion about boundaries or feelings. That's okay. You can opt to not do or say anything in the present moment. Sometimes "giving in" to what your family is asking of you is an act of self-preservation in the short term. That being said, think about both the short-term and long-term changes you hope to see. Be clear about what you feel is necessary to change right away versus what you are willing to accept will take time.

Sometimes they justify their actions with, "We don't talk about feelings." As with cultural and generational differences, sometimes you're not accustomed to discussing emotions and any "touchy-feely" subjects with people. Perhaps your parents have never spoken about these topics before and you can't even imagine what that would look like. Or maybe you've tried and you got such a negative reaction from them that you're not keen on revisiting that approach. In this case, how can you go about sharing what you need when there isn't that foundation or common language?

Start small and start with actions

People who aren't used to talking about deeper-rooted thoughts and feelings that underlie their relationship requests may be more inclined to want to discuss specific action items. It can be easier to approach your relationships by asking to see more of a specific behavior and for certain steps to be taken. When your parents keep making last-minute demands on your time, you feel stressed and overwhelmed, and you feel resentful that they don't respect your time. You may feel they're taking you for granted. You might not be able to say all of that, but you can turn it into a "do this instead" kind of request. This can sound like: "It's hard for me to plan my day when you drop last-minute requests. I want to help you, so I need you to ask me your favors at least two to three days in advance."

I know this may seem like a mind-blowing feat. "What do you mean, I'm going to tell my parents what to do?" I've seen clients gape when I've suggested potential ways they could change up their approach to these stressful situations. I gently challenge them, "Well, if this is something that's been making you feel resentful and frustrated for so long, then wouldn't you rather try to make things better?"

Remember, you get to tweak the approach in a way you think will lead to the ideal outcomes and suit your circumstances. The key here is to approach your relationships with a new attitude and mindset that you are allowed to have needs and you can learn how to share these with others.

It's not always a smooth ride: when people take issue with our new approach to relationships

I would be remiss if I didn't acknowledge the potential negative outcomes of speaking up for yourself. Sometimes people push back when we do something new. That pushback can come in different forms. When it comes in the form of gentle resistance, questioning, or discomfort, I still encourage you to stick with it. By continuing to assert yourself and incrementally practicing your active engagement strategies (like asking for help, stating an opinion or need, saying no), things can get better and feel easier over time. It makes sense that there will be some discomfort both within yourself and from others. It doesn't mean it's wrong. It just means it's new and something is changing. You're doing something to change patterns and it'll take time and practice to get used to it.

Perfectionistic people have to build up the strength to keep speaking up and asserting their feelings and needs. It's also an act of reasserting their voice. It can be exhausting. Asserting boundaries, especially when it's foreign to you, can feel like a lot of work. It's going to take some getting used to. Therefore it's crucial to have grace and patience with yourself as you learn this process of communicating your needs. Also, get outside support to help in your journey.

When enough is enough

You may fear being criticized, that others will get defensive or aggressive, or you will be ignored or rejected by speaking up. These are not ideal outcomes, so we need to be clear on what the difference is between being uncomfortable with change and being in a psychologically and emotionally damaging situation.

Sometimes it's not just about you getting used to change or merely a matter of time until other people will accept and adjust. Sometimes people are unwilling or unable to accept you for who you are and what you're trying to do to have a healthier relationship. The following are signs that there are larger, irreconcilable differences:

- repeated boundary violations
- constant criticism
- gaslighting
- abusive and toxic behaviors (verbal, financial, physical, emotional, social).

One of the common criticisms I hear come up when people try to speak up for how they feel is being told by others that they're "too sensitive." This is an example of gaslighting, a form of defensiveness on the part of the receiver of boundaries. Gaslighting is defined as "psychological manipulation of a person usually over an extended period of time that causes [someone] to question the validity of their own thoughts, perception of reality, or memories" (www.merriam-webster.com/dictionary/gaslighting). Examples of gaslighting statements include being told you're "too sensitive" or "too needy" for having said what you want or feel. Essentially, someone else is trying to make you feel that you're the problem for having said something when you provided feedback to the other person about their problematic behavior. This is like the client I spoke of earlier whose mother kept using her words against her and made her feel like a burden for having shared parts of herself.

A repeated lack of respect for your attempts to be yourself and have a say in the relationship is not okay. This is a "it's not you, it's them" situation. Truly. It's important to remember this can be an option, albeit an unfortunate one. Remember that not all situations are our responsibility to fix. Get some outside perspectives (i.e. from a therapist, trusted friends, family members) and then act accordingly. This can mean you end your communications with someone, distance yourself, or make an internal commitment to reallocate the amount of emotional and mental energy you'll expend on this person.

The key is not to blame yourself for having tried to make the relationship work and for whatever amount of time and resources you put into the relationship. We all do what we can with the information and good faith we have at the time. But as soon as you're more aware of what's going on and how you would like it to be different, you can take back control and make better decisions.

Yes, this is hard. Yes, this is normal

"I'm in my forties and yet it's so hard for me to speak up for myself. I thought I should know how to do this by now. It's embarrassing I can't stand up for myself to my parents at my age. Is this normal?"

I'm often asked why this is so hard for people and whether this is normal. I wholeheartedly and emphatically express a big *yes*. This is very normal. This is so common. It doesn't make things go away, but at the very least you can start to take off the pressure and self-judgment for having struggled with breaking problematic relationship patterns. It can be hard to break out of these ways of thinking because you've been reinforced to repeat these patterns. People encourage more of the same overdelivering, people-pleasing, and accommodating behaviors because those people/groups/systems benefit from you doing this.

People-pleasing proliferated throughout my life because I kept getting positive recognition, praise, and encouragement to do more. In our relationships, we're applauded by others for giving more of ourselves. You'll rarely be told "Please do less" or "Don't give me what I want." Since it's not necessarily going to come from others, it's important that you come to terms with the right to have limits and boundaries and then to know what those are for yourself and recognize when your limits have been reached.

Rethinking your approach to relationships as a perfectionist

Perfectionists need to learn how to adopt a more flexible approach towards their relationships. This means you can still be aware of what is appropriate in certain situations while applying different rules in other situations. For example, just because you learned that in your family gatherings you're not allowed to offer dissenting opinions doesn't mean you can't do so at your job. Or just because avoiding conflict was something you were told you must do "at all costs" early on doesn't mean you have to continue carrying this message in the present day.

Start giving yourself permission to have limits and boundaries. Name what your version of boundaries is for different situations. Build the self-awareness to know when those boundaries have been violated and how to remedy it.

Do the work of unlearning the outdated relationship shoulds. Adopt new relationship values that guide your approach to healthy relationships.

My identity as a perfectionist and people-pleaser was an asset in the sense that I learned how to blend in and do what was expected of me and to be acceptable to others. It helped me succeed academically and professionally. However, the constant self-monitoring and trying to be approved of and accepted according to others' standards hampered my self-knowing and confidence in who I was. I felt as though I lost the core of who I was and what I stood for. I didn't have a sense of what *I* truly wanted, not what the "perfect" version of myself learned she *should* want. Reckoning with this loss of myself meant I had to re-evaluate my values and build that core back up – reconstructing it with the things I wanted and valued. Later in the book you will find our foray into evaluating your values and tying those to the things you choose to do – whether they're at work or in your personal relationships. Getting clearer on those values can help turn your perfectionistic tendencies into superpowers.

New relationship values to abide by

- There is such a thing as healthy conflict.
- Vulnerability can strengthen relationships.
- Asking for what you want and need can lead to greater understanding and more satisfying relationships.
- Speaking up for yourself is an act of self-value and agency, not being "rude" and "selfish."
- Boundaries help build relationships based on mutual respect.
- There are times and places when certain "rules" fit and when they don't. You can determine this through practice and feedback.
- Relational mistakes will occur and that is okay. In the right types of relationships, you can repair them and build back stronger connections.

5
Embracing imperfection

Introduction

Imperfection gets a bad rep. When you hear the word "imperfect," what comes to mind?

- broken
- flawed
- unacceptable
- needing to be fixed
- wrong
- incomplete
- strange
- not good enough.

To curb our relationship to perfectionism, we need to value the imperfect nature of things. Imperfectionism, the counterpart to perfectionism, is the acceptance of imperfections as good enough and worthy of value. It's letting go of the limited views we hold, both as individuals and as a society, that imperfections are wrong and bad. When we're open to a new interpretation of imperfections, it opens us up to a world of possibilities. This is high praise for a concept that holds such a negative connotation. Imperfection can go from being something you fear and loathe to something you embrace and in some cases deem better than perfect.

This idea of embracing imperfection is not something I've made up. There are cultural, religious, and spiritual beliefs that are rooted in similar beliefs around imperfection. For example, "wabi-sabi" is a Japanese cultural aesthetic that appreciates the beauty in what is imperfect and impermanent. Also, consider what greater creators and thinkers from all disciplines—from technology, visual arts, and media to social justice and education—have done with imperfect, seemingly flawed things. They've been able to make more powerful and beautiful things with them. It started with them going beyond limited views of "perfection."

Adopting a different perspective about imperfection helps us be less judgmental and self-critical and it can help open us up to new experiences. This chapter is all about how to start embracing the "imperfectionist" in all of us.

Rethinking imperfection

Embracing imperfection helps us take more risks, embark on less certain paths, and make inroads into ventures we previously wanted to embark on but felt afraid of. Here is an incomplete list of the benefits of embracing imperfection:

- larger capacity to take risks, start and follow through with goals
- greater self-compassion
- more patience and empathy for ourselves and others
- increased flexibility and adaptability to new or challenging situations
- self-growth and learning from a place of curiosity
- higher resilience and tolerance for mistakes and failures
- having more life experiences because you're willing to try new things.

If I had to sum up all the benefits of embracing imperfection, it'd be this:

You will suffer far less in life and live more fully when you accept things as they are and stop trying to force things to be how they shouldn't be or forcing yourself to be someone you're not.

Given there are so many benefits to embracing imperfection, why do we struggle with it?

What's so wrong with imperfection?

Personally, it took me a long time to buy into the concept of accepting imperfection and practicing a "good enough" approach. It's hard for most of us because we have been taught that imperfections, flaws, and failures will lead to negative outcomes such as criticism and rejection. Perfectionism became a protective shield against experiencing things we fear, such as social disconnection, emotional exposure, and uncertain outcomes.

Fear of social disconnection and emotional exposure

We avoid anything that might risk us feeling rejected. We rely on our connections to others to survive and thrive. Perfectionism is one way of trying to guarantee our chances of being accepted into groups, forming close relationships, and feeling safe in society.

However, there is a difference between belonging and "fitting in." Most of the time we misinterpret fitting in with a real experience of belonging. When you're busy pleasing, and performing, and proving yourself through perfectionistic means, it's more in service of fitting in as opposed to belonging.

Vulnerability leads to genuine connections that evoke a real sense of belonging. Emotional exposure is one aspect of vulnerability. As we discussed in Chapter 4, perfectionists and people-pleasers avoid being vulnerable because they would rather be seen as "strong" and never expose "weak" emotions. However, relationships suffer when people can't ever bring themselves to be honest with their partners or friends about what they're going through.

Being honest looks like sharing imperfections in your life, such as the less-than-ideal circumstances you're currently experiencing, the messy emotions and thoughts you have, and the fact that you don't know everything.

My clients describe feeling ashamed when they admit, "I don't know what I'm doing," assuming they're alone in feeling this way. They judge themselves harshly because they believe being perfect means knowing everything. When they come to understand that being a real human being means having imperfect information and *not* having all of the answers, they feel a sense of liberation and relief. Even when you have some of life's answers, you may not always get situations "right" the first time around. Or the second or third. Accept that this process of making mistakes and feeling uncertain is a normal part of living and there is nothing wrong with you for going through this. The more you accept these experiences for yourself, the easier it will be to share these experiences with others. When others see you're willing to be vulnerable and expose these parts of yourself, they too will have an easier time expressing themselves.

The more we embrace imperfection, the more compassionate, accepting, and empathetic we become. We become less focused on judging ourselves so harshly to such unrealistic standards and by extension apply that same non-judgmental attitude towards others.

Fear of uncertainty

Avoiding uncertainty looks like avoiding risks, not speaking up, staying small, and forcing our control over things that don't lend themselves to being controlled (but we try so hard regardless!). As a result, we procrastinate on small to larger tasks/goals/dreams and engage in thought patterns like "what if," "if . . . then," "if only," and all-or-nothing thinking to delay and avoid action. The attempt to make things certain can explain why we suffer from anxiety, chronic stress, and depression. It can make us physically, emotionally, and mentally unwell when we put it on ourselves to try to control aspects of life that aren't ours to control.

We fear what we think will be negative and what we assume is "bad." This means we *think* in certain ways that reinforce this notion that there is indeed a clear good and bad. In this case, we *think* perfection is the good thing to strive for while imperfection is bad and should be avoided. Next, let's talk about *how* we're thinking and consider maybe there are alternatives.

Thought patterns that keep us stuck

"If only" thinking is the pattern of second guessing how you did something and considering you could have done something better.

- "If only I had spent more time on this, then I would've gotten it perfect."
- "If only I act more like the people at work, then I'll get promoted."

Similarly, **"if . . . then" thinking** is based on the assumption that you have to wait for something else to happen before you get to experience something else.

- "If I make more money, then I'll be happy."

"What if" thinking shows up as spending more time deliberating the potential outcomes rather than taking steps towards something. This comes from feeling the need to prepare for all potential scenarios before taking action.

- "What if I fail?"
- "What if I say something stupid and she rejects me?"
- "What if I tell my boss no and then they'll think I'm lazy and I get fired?"

"Black-and-white" thinking, also described as all-or-nothing thinking or dichotomous thinking, is when you lump things into just two categories, such as good or bad, perfect or failure. Perfectionists often operate under black-and-white thinking. This is where unrealistic, extreme, and/or rigid standards come from.

In certain situations, black-and-white thinking can be helpful. We don't want to deliberate about all of the possible options when we're trying to problem solve, come up with practical solutions, and take deliberate action steps. "This versus that" is helpful when making judgments about which grocery store items to get, or which tax service to employ to help you file your annual taxes. But when it comes to more human-centered choices, about features of our daily lives that are filled with nuance and are context-specific, this black-and-white thinking is less useful. Black-and-white thinking fails to take into account life circumstances, context, dynamic relationships, and the fact that we're constantly evolving, emotional, and for better or worse, unpredictable.

Expanding our ways of thinking

We need to adopt a more flexible and expansive way of thinking that goes beyond the "what ifs," the good versus bad, and "if . . . then" hypotheticals. Rather than make it about good versus bad, or success versus failure, make room for a spectrum of possibilities. It's unrealistic to ask you to avoid making judgments since we're constantly having to make assessments and decisions, so instead practice a process-oriented approach when you assess a situation. Let's look at an example.

In the beginning stages of a new hobby, ask:

• "How does this feel as I'm *starting* this new thing?"

As you move further along in the process of this hobby, ask:

• "How have I been changing over time?"

Near the end of the process, ask:

• "What have I learned so far?"

Finally, at the end, ask:

• "What did I learn?"
• "What am I proud of?"
• "What surprised me?"
• "When I do something like this again, what would I do differently?"

Use open-ended questions for a better understanding of your feelings, for surprises and changes, and to appreciate the nuanced aspects of your experience. With practice, you can get better at recognizing in which situations to apply these different ways of thinking.

Cognitive dissonance

Cognitive dissonance happens when there's a mismatch between our thoughts and the outcomes of our behaviors. As perfectionists, when we feel cognitive dissonance, our initial impulse is to "fix" what we think is wrong by changing our behaviors. What underlies this impulse to fix is our desire to reset ourselves to a place of emotional congruence and out of what we think is a "bad" place.

Remember, dissonance exists because we have a certain *thought* about how things "should" be. When things don't meet that standard, we think things are wrong and see them in a negative light. But what if we could change our original interpretation? Rather than immediately thinking, "Oh no, this is bad/wrong/unacceptable," what if we could think, "This is interesting/acceptable/enough" or "This is something to learn from and work with"? Changing our thought patterns like this is a type of expansive thinking.

When we're able to change our interpretations of an outcome, we can change our feelings about it too. It neutralizes that dissonance. It can even shift it into a positive experience. That's the power of taking a more curious, open-minded approach to the things we see. Breaking predefined notions of what is "right" away from the unrealistic standard of perfect, and instead allowing things to be as they are, can be incredibly liberating. When you're no longer immediately shutting down at the first sign of imperfection, you're probably going to feel less stressed and critical of yourself.

This shift towards a more curious and open stance regarding imperfection will lead to more creative solutions, better outcomes, and enjoyable processes. Speaking of processes, learning to embrace imperfection is a process and will take some relearning of old messages and redefining what we see as "good enough."

Accepting good enough

If perfectionism is rooted in our unrealistically high standards, embracing imperfection means we allow some things to meet *good enough* standards. Accepting good enough can change both how we'll go about doing things and our expectations of the outcomes. Perfectionists fall into the trap of trying to constantly optimize things, even at the risk of making things harder for themselves. As we discussed before, perfectionists think the "right" way to do things is by themselves, by any means necessary. They can take the "hard" in "hard work" a step too far. All of this overfunctioning and striving towards unrealistic standards can lead to burnout, shutting down, and dissatisfaction in your life and your relationships. Therefore, adopting a more flexible mindset that allows for "good enough," including imperfections along the way, will relieve the pressure we put on ourselves. It might even help you ultimately get to the ideal outcome with the bonus of not straining yourself in the process.

What is "good enough"?

The phrase "good enough" can feel difficult for perfectionists to stomach because we're taught that bigger and better are the things to strive for. What's the sense in being "good enough" when there's always something better? Our culture is obsessed with optimization and making "the best choice" in a world of endless options. This makes choosing "good enough" difficult.

There is a misconception that good enough means you're settling for less-than and mediocre results. But good enough does not have to mean you're settling. It can mean you're going to choose in advance what is important to you and define specifically how you'd like to get there. It can mean you're more focused on actually experiencing something and going along for the ride rather than searching for how to do it or what is better. Here are some things to look out for to accept what is good enough.

- Find a new, specific metric for "good enough" or "your best." Redefine this in different terms, such as how valuable it is, how this makes things easier for you and/or others, how this contributes to your larger goals and a greater purpose.
- Focus on the process, not just the outcome. Be thoughtful about what you'd like to get out of this experience, not just what you think you'll achieve at the end.
- Get clear on what matters most. Accept that making a choice and taking action will require tradeoffs. Tradeoffs are neutral and necessary.

Let's say you're starting to reach a point where you're into this whole idea of good enough. But what does that actually mean in practice? It means moving it a step further into the realm of taking some risks and becoming comfortable with being uncomfortable. When we're willing to *grow* outside of perfectionistic bounds, there are inherently some risks we're going to take and uncertainty to be had. Building emotional resilience will help with our ability to tolerate risk, mistakes, and uncertainty.

Taking risks: it's the start of something new

I often hear perfectionists describe themselves as "risk-averse." This means they would prefer not to approach situations or pursue things that seem risky. They assume risky means dangerous, so it would make sense to avoid such options. Perfectionists prefer to know all of the details and feel ready and prepared before taking steps. This is their attempt to avoid failure and other outcomes they perceive as negative.

Notice I say "perceive as negative." This means not all negative outcomes are as bad as we think they are. It is important to know the difference between negative outcomes to avoid because they will harm ourselves and others versus negative outcomes to avoid because they're new and force us to grapple with uncertainty. Obviously, we want to avoid the former. A certain degree of thoughtfulness and intentionality is wise. However, avoiding the latter can hamper your ability to grow and experience a richer life.

Avoidance can show up in a lot of different ways, even some well-meaning behaviors like researching and overpreparing for a plan of action. It takes time for people to feel ready to change and to take those first steps, but how much time is too much time?

Rabbit holes: stages of change

When it comes to starting something new, I have a certain process. I will usually write about it for some time to get more comfortable with the idea. Once I wrap my head around it, I embark on finding as many answers to my questions as I can. I do a lot of research, listen to people in similar situations, and gather as much advice as I possibly can about how to do something and what I can expect. The amount of time I stay in what I'll call the "research phase" can vary from a few days to many weeks and sometimes months. Sound familiar?

In psychology, the Transtheoretical Stages of Change model describes a series of stages that people move through when it comes to making changes in behavior patterns and habits. The stages are:

1 Pre-contemplation.
2 Contemplation.
3 Preparation.

4 Action – the biggest stumbling block for perfectionists.
5 Maintenance.

When people get caught in the trap of rabbit holes of information gathering and planning, they're essentially stuck in the stages of contemplation and preparation.

If you're like me, you might be stuck in that place for much longer than is helpful. You're avoiding moving onto the next stage: action.

What we're avoiding when we avoid action

Action means we're on the hook for the thing we want. Action means we will put something out into the world. We're not exactly sure what will happen, but we know we're going to open ourselves to some sort of reaction. Reactions can range from external – making mistakes, things not going as smoothly as you thought, negative or positive feedback – to internal – self-judgment, self-doubt, pride, disappointment, surprise. The uncertainty over how it's going to go is enough to make us stay stuck in that preparation place. We engage in a kind of magical thinking that maybe, if we just look into one more option or wait a little longer, we will ensure the best possible outcome.

Think of all of the times you stopped yourself from taking the first step towards something you wanted to try because the thought of it *not* going well felt like too much.

"Don't you think it's too risky? Are you sure?"

"What about this, or that, or what if what if what if?"

The "what if's" can be endless.

Each time we give into those fear-driven thoughts around risks, we reinforce this pattern of avoidance. When we respond to the voice inside us that says "Don't do it! It's too scary!" and avoid taking that first step, the voice temporarily recedes into the background. For a moment, we feel relief. "Phew, crisis averted. Good thing you didn't try that awful idea!" But this keeps us stuck and still fearing something that has not happened. Our fear of things possibly being imperfect gets in the way of growing. To grow, we must accept that there will be some uncomfortable moments. We need to learn to trust that we can move through them and that what's on the other side is worth the risk.

Undoing to get unstuck

Growth is a non-linear, upward, spiral-like process. Think of it as the good kind of spiral. Rather than spiraling downward into negative thoughts and avoidance behaviors, openness to imperfect action and risk-taking can lead to upward spirals of growth.

People get stuck and don't grow when they stop at the first sign of challenge. At the first sign of something being "imperfect," aka broken, wrong, incorrect, or hard, people will balk and turn around. They won't try again, they'll revert to something old, or they'll make up some story about why this is something they don't care about. Perfectionists have a low tolerance for these challenging moments. They might be able to persist through them, but internally, if they interpret these challenges as something wrong with them, they won't really learn the benefits of the challenges. They'll only use the challenge as one more thing they need to fix, not as something they can learn from.

We have to accept setbacks as a means of growth. Not everything will work the first time. Sometimes you have to back up and try a new approach to make progress towards your ultimate goal. Starting over or having to retrace your steps doesn't have to be seen as wrong. Instead, these are necessary steps in the growth process.

No one wrote a perfect piece of music or novel in one sitting without having revised it or looked at it again with different ears or eyes. It required changes. Changes don't have to be the be-all and end-all to something we're attempting to create. Instead, it's a normal part of the process of creating. Similarly, we need to see our lives as a constant process of creating experiences. We're going to make mistakes along the way, whether it's in the way we speak to someone, how we go about trying something new at work or in our personal lives, or something as simple as cooking a dish. It's important to normalize these steps of going over something again and approaching things differently.

We have to learn how to accept a certain degree of uncertainty and let things remain gray and ambiguous. Not everything is built to be black and white. We don't know everything and we won't know everything. Some things can be left unknown. A lot of suffering comes from our attempts to force the gray to be black and white or to make the uncertain certain.

Steps to help you move towards action

Ask yourself: *What's holding me back? Where do I tend to get hung up when I consider starting something new? When do I tend to get stuck?*

- Are you an overthinker? Do you stay in the Contemplation phase for a long time?
- Do you stay in the Preparation phase? Do you get stuck doing a lot of research?

- Do you make endless lists of options and considerations before making a decision?
- Do you watch others do what you wish you could do and simply leave it at that?
- Are you overly comfortable in dreaming and ideating about something you *could* do or wish was possible?

The Contemplation phase is a creative space, but you can't afford to stay there forever. Remember, your goal is to get something done or to experience something new. If you're someone who gets drawn into creating and ideating (Contemplation phase), make a list of the next action-oriented steps you need to take to get the idea of what you want from an abstract wish, idea, or intention to a concrete plan. Make things look, feel, and sound more real.

> Example: "I would love to be someone who can feel more comfortable speaking in public settings" to "I will look at public speaking classes that are available to me. I will ask my friends for recommendations. I will look at my schedule to see when I will carve out time for this open mic event where I can watch people I admire. I want to see models of people who can show me what taking risks can look like and how fun it can be."

Overpreparers tend to overdo the lists and planning (Preparation phase), so designate a point where enough is enough. If your gauge of what is enough tends to be off (in other words, you struggle to ever let things go), then rally someone else's perspective and support. This is where a bit of tough love and accountability will help.

Those who struggle with analysis-paralysis and have trouble making decisions should set limits through techniques such as setting timers for immediate lower-stakes decisions and deadlines for shorter- to longer-term goals and decisions. Both limits and boundaries can be used to your advantage when your tendency is to let things go on for too long.

Address the self-doubts and voices that keep you from being an active participant in your own endeavors. Rather than just dreaming of what could be or watching others do the things you dream of, confront what is holding you back from believing *you* can be the one to have these things. This could be a matter of not knowing what's the next immediate step, it can be because you have doubts about your ability to follow through, or it can be the fear of making mistakes. Whatever those beliefs or questions may be, address them. Don't let them linger and keep you stuck.

Build up your risk tolerance. Once we succeed in small acts of risk-taking in low-stakes situations, we'll be more willing to do it again. We can repeat these behaviors and extend them to other areas of our lives that can have an even greater impact on our lives. Start as small as you need, but make an honest attempt at that small step. This is the way to quiet that knee-jerk reaction that says, "Are you sure?" You can prove to yourself that you trust yourself and that it is not dangerous.

Rally the support of other people. We rarely can get through things by ourselves. Talk to someone you trust and have them support you through this process. Maybe they can do something with you or help you overcome hurdles getting in your way. Share your progress of taking small risks with others and reward yourself along the way. This can be as small as acknowledging your first step by saying to yourself, "I'm proud of myself for finally trying this."

Write affirmations and reminders to yourself that help combat the voice that has tried to stop you from taking steps before. Gently talk back to the inner voice of doubt and fear that pops up with those "what if?" questions. Change it from an unquestioned monologue to a constructive dialogue. Brené Brown once shared that before she enters new situations, she tells herself, "I am not here to be right. I am here to get it right" (www.linkedin.com/pulse/transcript-episode-101-bren%C3%A9-brown-getting-right-jessi-hempel/).

The antidote to fear: curiosity and mindfulness

Curiosity is a powerful antidote to old black-and-white thinking and fear. When something goes from "What if?" and a limiting belief that things have to be a certain way to "Why not?" and "What else is possible here?" and a more expansive belief that imperfections could be an opportunity for growth, things feel a lot lighter. A curious attitude towards life makes things a little less intimidating and invites a greater sense of possibility.

Mindfulness is the practice of observing things in the present moment with a non-judgmental attitude. You're essentially letting things be as they are rather than labeling them as good or bad. When you can let go of the tendency to judge everything through such a critical lens, you can stop thinking of everything as a problem to be fixed. Mindfulness helps you slow down and practice distancing yourself from your constant barrage of thoughts, and the inner and outer noise of perfectionism, expectations, and societal pressure.

Here are some mindfulness-based strategies that will help you slow down and adopt this curious mindset that allows for imperfections just as they are, not as things to be fixed and controlled.

- **Get out of your head and into your body.** Perfectionists tend to be very cerebral and rational. They think through all of the ways they need to get it right. Being so calculated and cautious can lead to someone staying in their head with the risk of not being able to experience the present moment. Embodied activities such as physical movement, art, spending time in leisure activities alone or with people all help us connect back to our bodies.
- **Return to the present moment.** Thinking about the past and the future can keep us away from the present moment. There is a lot of advice out there to "smell the roses" and I know it's tempting to roll your eyes at this, but there is a reason that phrase won't go away. Notice when your mind is going to the past or planning for the future. If it's not necessary to plan something, see if you can afford to return your attention to what's going on now. "What am I feeling right now?" Take stock of basic sensory information to help you come back to now (what you smell, hear, taste, hear, and see).
- **Slow down and simplify.** Our fast-paced world is filled with constant stimulation and messages to hustle, move quickly, and do more. This makes it hard to slow down and consider how we're feeling and experiencing things. Literally, slow down how you're moving your body, prioritize one thing at a time, and reduce the number of distractions in your environment.

Overall, embracing imperfection opens us up to much more than what we've come to believe is "good." Embracing imperfection means allowing all of the humanity in us to have a place in our lives. Imperfections exist as a reminder of how things simply can be. We can choose to accept things as they are and be okay with it. We can choose to accept our *imperfect selves* as we are. In our culture of constant growth and self-improvement, that can sound like a ridiculous proposition. It's a necessary departure from all of the striving we have become accustomed to doing. It is radical. Radical acceptance of imperfect and good enough can be an essential part of living a life of more ease.

6
Living beyond perfectionism

Introduction

My foray into better understanding perfectionism wasn't academic. It wasn't even clinical. It was personal. When I came across so many other people who were struggling to see themselves beyond who they were as "perfectionists," I felt it was important to share my story. I *feel* as though it's a personal and political responsibility of mine to help others to overcome the barriers that hold us back from embracing a life above and beyond perfectionism.

This chapter is about the "other" parts of us that exist beyond perfectionism. We want to get more familiar with the multiple facets of our identity, not just the perfectionist. We are perfectionists *and* more.

I hope this provides you with a sense of hope and optimism. It's one thing to learn why we've become this way, meaning people who strive so hard to be perfect and achieve success according to internalized standards and expectations. It's another thing to also learn to accept how your perfectionistic ways have served a useful purpose in your life. Perfectionism is not necessarily something we have to get rid of. I shared earlier that I don't believe perfectionism, like so many other traits, is something we "cure" or a trait that will go away completely. Instead, I believe perfectionism will continue to play some role in our lives – the only issue is whether you'll let it take over completely or not. You can live with perfectionism without being taken over by it. Rather, the attributes we commonly associate with perfectionism, such as people-pleasing, being achievement-oriented, and holding high standards, can co-exist and function well with others.

When we let go of perfectionism being the gold standard of living and embrace imperfection, we can live more fully in the other parts. We can round out all of these traits and behaviors and have them be rooted in our values so that they work harmoniously.

The good behind perfectionism

I've gone through many examples of how perfectionism gone rampant and unexamined can have downsides for many aspects of our well-being. But just as there are downsides, there are also upsides. In Chapter 2 we explored the origins of perfectionism and the larger reasons these tendencies grew and continued throughout our lives. Perfectionism has served a positive function in our lives. For example, it helped you reach goals, accomplish things you're proud of, and maintain positive relationships. I want you to remain proud of those accomplishments. At the same time, I want you to have a more realistic expectation of how far being perfectionistic can take you and the potential opportunity costs of leaning so far into perfectionism.

Being mindful of the degree or timing of when we're "in that part" of ourselves will help minimize the risk of overdoing it and reaching that unhealthy level of perfectionism that makes things worse. What do I mean by perfectionism being a "part" of yourself with which you can develop this healthier relationship?

Perfectionism as a part

If you imagine the whole of your being like a family, then the traits, interests, and qualities of your personality are characters of that family. I'm sure you can think of times when members of your family acted adversarially or when they coexisted harmoniously. Certain members may have been struggling, so others had to step up to pick up the emotional or physical slack. Or members may have experienced a period of working in sync to elevate one another during times of stress or joy, which contributed to the feeling that things were fitting well in the grand scheme of life.

Think of perfectionism as one of these parts of your family of traits. You developed this perfectionistic part for a reason. You might have needed to more firmly control your situation, perform to high standards to get approval, and be "perfect" to smooth things out. The combination of your own needs and the societal approval of these behaviors reinforced that part. The perfectionistic part emerged as a larger, more heavily relied upon character. It made up for those parts of you that felt lacking and thus didn't get paid any attention. You may have felt certain traits were unnecessary or were hindrances to achieving success, approval, and security.

Using this "parts" language has helped me and many others work with aspects of their identity, personality traits, strengths, and weaknesses. Psychologically, using this model helps people work towards greater acceptance of the various parts of themselves, especially the parts that feel harder to accept. It doesn't help to judge any part of ourselves harshly or to disparage ourselves for being "this way."

Start with an attitude of curiosity. Use the following reflection prompts to help you see the good in the perfectionistic part.

Reflection questions: the good in perfectionism

- Think of instances in the past week when perfectionism helped you.
- Think of examples in the past year when perfectionism helped you.
- How have your perfectionistic qualities helped you get to where you are today?
- What are some things you appreciate about being a perfectionist?

Notice how reflecting upon perfectionism with a curious attitude helps you shift towards greater acceptance and understanding of the many ways it has helped you. This shift in thinking is a process and it's not always easy to re-examine parts of ourselves with a different attitude. So if you catch yourself judging the perfectionistic part, try reminding yourself with phrases such as:

Perfectionism played a useful purpose in my life in the past.

Perfectionism helped me get through life/difficult circumstances/overcome obstacles/succeed to the degree I needed to.

I appreciate that being a perfectionist was something necessary in my life at certain times.

My perfectionist part is just one part of who I am.

I will patiently work towards accepting perfectionism as a helpful part of my life.

Too much of a good thing

"I get that it helped me in the past, but it still feels like perfectionism controls me and makes me more miserable."

As we know with other experiences in life, there can be such a thing as too much of a good thing. When perfectionism can get to be too much, we experience the negative effects on our mental, physical, and social health (e.g. relationship problems, burnout, loss of identity). This unhealthy level of perfectionism is often a result of a lack of conscious awareness of how it's functioning in our lives. This means that perfectionistic behaviors and thought patterns have become habits and operate in autopilot mode. When anything becomes that automatic and out of our conscious awareness, it runs the risk of being overused.

How do we stop this from happening? Building self-awareness is one of the necessary and powerful first steps before change can happen. We can't accept something we're not even aware is happening, much less change it.

How to keep the perfectionism in check

Give the perfectionist part a job

Give it a title with a specific role it plays in your life. Writer Anne Lamott calls her part the "Ethical Consultant" (podcast interview, "Anne Lamott: Make your writing fears work for YOU," The Screen Writing Life with Meg LeFauve and Lorien McKenna). When it's time to judge a certain situation and she wants to use the high, scrutinizing standards so characteristic of perfectionism, she'll call upon the Ethical Consultant to guide her decisions.

Remember, perfectionism doesn't always need to be present in certain situations. Just like some members of your family don't get invited to specific events, you can choose not to extend the invitation of perfectionism. "Not now" is something you can say.

Take a Goldilocks Method to perfectionistic standards

It's not wrong to have standards that you want to achieve. Having too few or vague standards can look like having no values, no standard of living and operating in life, being wishy-washy, or as though you're lacking a moral or ethical compass. Having too many leads to being hypercritical, judgmental, chronically stressed, irritable, and unable to control the standards' hold on you. The Goldilocks Method means you find metrics or standards that are just right.

Redefine what good enough looks like in specific terms. You can practice this using phrases such as "this is enough," "good enough," and "for now." These phrases relieve the perfectionistic pressure to overdo or become overburdened by unrealistic expectations. Feel free to add these and your own Goldilocks versions of "good enough" to your vocabulary.

Use mindfulness and self-reflection questions

Mindfulness increases the degree of conscious awareness of your perfectionistic habits. Mindfulness is the act of intentionally paying attention with a non-judgmental attitude to an experience you're having in the present moment. Being aware of the "present moment" can take the form of:

- taking a walk outside
- taking a shower where you can decompress and have some time to yourself
- journaling
- talking things out with someone
- participating in a formal meditation session (e.g. silently sitting/laying down, undistracted and uninterrupted, guided or unguided practice)
- concentrating on your breath for a given amount of time and noticing the physical sensations that emerge.

The following questions can help you get a better handle on what is happening in the present moment and ultimately consider ways you can support yourself in the most helpful way possible. I have included specific questions aimed at questioning whether perfectionism is the necessary and most helpful part in a given situation.

- What kinds of emotions and thoughts are you experiencing right now?
- What sensations are you noticing in your body?
- What do you need right now?
- What urges are you currently having? Why might you be feeling the urge to act/say/think this way?
- Are you trying to avoid something? Are you afraid of a negative outcome?
- What is the outcome you're looking to achieve?
- Is this a situation where perfectionism is necessary? What are different ways you could get a similar outcome or experience without resorting to the perfectionistic part?
- What are other parts of yourself you can call upon to help achieve a similar outcome or get help with how you're feeling?

You can apply this model of self-examination to help accept any other trait or part in you, not just perfectionism. In fact, after you've done this with perfectionism, I invite you to think about other parts of yourself that you may have a hard time accepting (e.g. the part that finds it difficult to let go of grudges, the part that feels the need to control everything, the anxious part).

Building self-awareness and greater acceptance of the perfectionist part in you is a great start. But I also want you to think beyond just perfectionism. Given perfectionism is just one part, what other parts exist? Who are you beyond being a perfectionist?

Who are you? Your identity beyond the perfectionist

People struggle to let go of their identities as perfectionists, people-pleasers, or high achievers because they're not sure if they can identify other traits they're proud of or that have been recognized by others. So much of the work of reducing the outsized role perfectionism plays in your life is in paying closer attention to the other aspects of your identity that have been long unnoticed and underappreciated.

In many social situations, people focus too much attention on their job titles. Perfectionism can lead to becoming so hyper-focused on delivering on external expectations that people lose sight of what other internal traits and aspects of their identity have to offer. Remember, all parts have some value, so it's not about belittling any parts. Sometimes people struggle with giving themselves permission to claim parts of their identity because of assumptions about what makes it "real."

For example, when I started digging deeper into this identity-based work, I had a hard time claiming that I was "a creative." I didn't feel I had a right to claim it as a part of myself since I wasn't making visual art or doing things I deemed "real creatives" did. This is just another extension of perfectionism at play, letting my preconceived beliefs and unrealistic standards about what is "real" get in the way of accepting something I want. Similarly, I know people who struggle to claim they're an activist because their involvement in activism doesn't look like the public-facing activism they see in the media or how other people get involved in it.

You have a right to claim parts of yourself and name them in whatever way you want. These are deeply personal and there is no right or wrong in however you designate those parts. Here's another opportunity to practice in imperfect terms, thinking more expansively as opposed to in black-and-white terms about what is or isn't "right."

Use these prompts to identify yourself in various ways. These leave room to think about yourself in terms outside of your job title. You can identify by your strengths, your relationship roles, your passions, your hobbies, and your personality traits. Play with whatever language suits you. You can even describe yourself as a shade of a color, for example.

I am a . . .

I am passionate about . . .

I am into . . .

I like . . .

I love . . .

I dream of . . .

Relearning what is "right" for you

We have spent our lifetimes internalizing messages about what is worthwhile and what is deemed worthless. This includes prioritizing productivity over rest, work over play, valuing thinking over intuition or emotions, efficiency over joy, and self over community. By engaging in this black-and-white thinking, we devalue certain activities and things in life. Often those are devalued by systems and people who don't necessarily have our best interest in mind. It's time to rethink how much *we* value them, which is a process of relearning or deconditioning if you will.

Relearning is an active ongoing process. It takes work to get to know yourself as you are, not as others want you to be. This is an invitation to engage in some exercises that will get you going on the path to relearning the parts of who you are beyond being a perfectionist. You can do this through reflection exercises (such as the ones in this book), therapy, conversations with close friends, and learning from role models and teachers.

We will start with identifying your values. Next, we'll see how you can begin to better align your current life circumstances with your values. Ultimately, these exercises will help give some clarity about how you want to live and direct your actions towards living a more values-aligned life.

This may be the first time you are sitting down to answer questions such as these. For many of my clients, therapy is one of the first and rare opportunities where this kind of self-inquiry is taking place. Here are a few pieces of advice:

- Be patient with yourself.
- Be mindful of *how* you're even going through these exercises.
- Don't feel the need to have an answer to questions right away. Take your time, do it in chunks if needed, and do it when you have the mental and emotional bandwidth.
- Invite another person to join you.

Ultimately, I want you to do what works for you.

What do you stand for? Identifying your values

One of the reasons you might struggle to feel a sense of purpose and meaning in your life is because the things you're doing don't fit with what you truly care about and desire. Perfectionism can mask your true desires because one of the pursuits of perfectionists is to meet the expectations of others.

This is why the constant pursuit of other people's goals isn't all that fulfilling in the long run. Goals we try to achieve that aren't rooted in our values can feel meaningless. We only get the short-term reward of having achieved some outcome.

However, it won't feed that deeper part of yourself that wants to experience something meaningful to you. Therefore, we need to be aware of what our values are and then let those guide the decisions we make about how we spend our time, who we spend our time with and for, and what we'll choose to leave out of our lives and say no to.

Exercise: Defining your values

Look at the list in the values table and then decide on three value words that mean the most to you in defining what you stand for and that guide your decisions and priorities.

Values table

Acceptance	Environment	Justice	Play
Accountability	Ethics	Kindness	Recognition
Achievement	Excellence	Knowledge	Respect
Adaptability	Exploration	Leadership	Responsibility
Adventure	Fairness	Learning	Risk-taking
Ambition	Family	Leisure	Self-actualization
Assertiveness	Financial stability	Love	Service
Authenticity	Freedom	Loyalty	Simplicity
Balance	Friendship	Mastery	Solitude
Belonging	Fun	Maturity	Spirituality
Beauty	Health	Meaning	Stability
Caring	Honesty	Nature	Status

Clarity	Humility	Novelty	Structure
Community	Humor	Openness	Teamwork
Compassion	Independence	Order	Thoughtfulness
Courage	Innovation	Originality	Time
Creativity	Integrity	Passion	Trust
Curiosity	Intelligence	Patience	Uniqueness
Discipline	Intuition	Peace	Vulnerability
Diversity	Joy	Perseverance	Wisdom

Write your own:

The instructions are simple, but in execution it's not always so easy. Your goal is to ultimately land on no more than three. Why three? I am a firm believer that when we claim to abide by too many values, it muddies what we really stand for. It diminishes the importance of the values that are supposed to be our guiding lights.

Here are some tips to help with the narrowing-down process:

- Start with a larger group of 5–10 values that stick out to you.
- Take time away from the list. Return and assess which ones out of the 5–10 move closer to the top in terms of importance and salience.
- Repeat this iterative process of pausing, coming back, and noting the ones that are more important than the others until you've landed on the three.

At the end of the day, it's more important that you're doing the exercise of thinking through what is meaningful to you and what drives a life you find worth living. Remember, this is very personal and customized to you. It's not the time to have a perfectionistic approach to this exercise. Heaven forbid, this is even a bit fun!

Values in action

Values are not just "what I care about" or "things I like." If that was all they were, they'd simply be aspirational traits, not much else. Or as Brené Brown says, "Values without action . . . become a joke. A cat poster. Total BS."

When you are clear about what these values look like in practice, you can make intentional decisions about how to spend your time and where to direct your attention. You will also be able to detect when you're not in internal alignment with those values and have a sense of how to course-correct.

Exercise: Operationalizing your values

Take a look at your values and create a list of as many as 5–10 behaviors that support those values. They can be things you are currently doing or example behaviors that will support your values. For example, one of my values is "learning." I view myself as a lifelong student. In action, behaviors that support this value are:

1 I invest my time and resources in activities that help me expand my worldview, experience new things, and learn something. Specifically, I go to museums regularly, check out books from the library, and attend lectures by writers, speakers, and other creatives, especially those who are not in my field.
2 I donate to programs and organizations that promote learning or education, broadly speaking.

The importance of living in alignment with your values

Whether you want to call it living according to your values or "living your best life," it all has to do with our human desire for coherence. When there is a misalignment between what we care about and what we're doing, we feel a sense of dis-ease, a different type of cognitive dissonance. I hear people describe this as feeling disingenuous, disconnected, inauthentic, as though they're not living up to their potential, or not sure if they know who they are. They say things like:

- "Something just doesn't feel right."
- "I'm going through the motions of my life, but that's all. What I do doesn't feel that meaningful to me. I feel like I'm running through someone's agenda."
- "I feel empty even though I'm supposedly doing all of the 'right' things."
- "Is this all there is to my life? I feel like there should be more."

In addition to discovering new parts of our identity, I believe we should celebrate parts that already exist. Some of us have been conditioned to overlook or denigrate certain parts of ourselves, maybe because we were told they were problematic or "too much."

- What are the personality traits that you struggle to accept?
- What are some things you used to be interested in that have taken a back seat because of trying to be perfect, trying to please other people?

  Have you considered what it would be like to reclaim those traits, supposed "weaknesses," and let them have a bigger say in how you live your life? What could that look like in practice? How would it feel to accept those parts of yourself?

Exercise: Auditing your current way of life

Use this exercise to audit how you're doing currently in terms of living in alignment with your values.

1 Look at your schedule. If you don't formally keep one, write down the events of a typical week with the activities you engage in.
2 Write down a list of the people you tend to spend the most time with or stay in contact with throughout a week.
3 You may even look at your recent expenses, which can sometimes serve as another source of information about what you consider to be major priorities.
4 After looking at your schedule, list of people, and where your resources go, ask yourself:
   – How do I feel about the way I'm spending my time, relationships, and money?
   – What do I love spending time and energy doing?
   – Where do I wish I spent less time and energy?
5 Take a look at your values and the values-in-action (list of behaviors). Use these to guide the following step.
6 Put a "+" sign for areas where you would like to invest more time and energy because they're aligned with your values and operationalized behaviors. Put a "–" sign next to the areas where you want to invest less time and energy because they don't align with your values.

Looking forward

It's very normal to see gaps between what you say you value and what you're currently doing. You won't be alone in this. We don't often take such a formal approach to assessing our everyday behaviors. Consider these misaligned areas of your life as workable. You have the information to inform the next steps you can take to get closer to living a life aligned with your values.

- List some action steps you can take to further cultivate and live into those values.
- Use the prompt "The kind of person I want to be" and write down some aspirations about the sorts of behaviors that will help you become that kind of person. An example is, "I want to be the kind of person who maintains valuable relationships. This means I will follow through on my commitments and say no to requests on my time that take away from those valuable relationships."
- Reflect and re-evaluate regularly. This will keep you accountable. Also, you want to make room for normal circumstances shifting in life and remain adaptable. If and when you stray from acting within your values, know you can always course-correct.
- Embed yourself in a community of others who celebrate similar values or will support you in living in alignment with yours.

All in all, this work of reflecting, defining specific behaviors, and taking deliberate action moves you towards the purpose of living the life you want to live.

Living a values-aligned life

By living aligned with your values, you learn to appreciate the little things in life. You can experience more gratitude and a sense of wonder, awe, and joy for the small things when you're not so mired in the details of your daily to-do list or feeling so down due to pressure. You have more emotional and mental space to appreciate things you didn't notice before.

My clients who started to invest in other parts of their lives outside of work or obligatory tasks shared that they were having more fun, getting to rest, had better physical health, and felt more emotionally stable. They began investing in old relationships and hobbies and discovered some new ones. They experienced getting closer to people in old and new relationships by being willing to be vulnerable and share. This was far more fulfilling when they felt a deeper sense of understanding and connection as opposed to the more guarded and shallow relationships they had before. Many of my clients started doing things "just because" to experiment with how it felt to embrace imperfection. It was fun to see them pick up random activities that were simply for the point of experiencing pleasure or learning something new.

The overfunctioner, Gabby, whom we met in Chapter 1, was able to practice setting boundaries between her work life and her personal life. While she previously couldn't imagine saying no to people's requests, she came to learn that saying no in a kind but firm manner could maintain her good working relationships, help her do her job well, and leave her with the mental and physical bandwidth at the end of a work day to enjoy her life outside of work. She shared, "I didn't realize that by saying yes to everything, I was overextending myself and making myself less effective in so many areas of my life. I can function at a more realistic capacity and still live into my values like being hardworking, considerate, and creative." She tapped more into the creative side of herself that she'd lost sight of by letting work override her schedule. With this spark in creativity, she felt more like a fuller version of herself, not the overrun overfunctioning workaholic.

Steven, who had struggled to see himself beyond being a chronic "lazy" procrastinator, did the inner work of letting go of the shame messaging he'd internalized for so long. He practiced taking small risks. One of those risks was giving himself permission to let small wins count. Giving himself credit for the small steps was so important to increase his sense of self-worth and confidence. He discovered how much he enjoyed the feedback of taking small actions and getting things done. Two of his values were adventure and community. He joined a climbing gym and met a great group of friends with whom he could practice challenging courses. There he described feeling "no judgment" for the mistakes and falls he'd make. He started referring to himself as a "good enough doer" – a far cry from the "lazy, unmotivated" person he'd previously considered himself to be.

Kai reached a place of burnout at her job where she was treated like a "pushover." She had internalized the message from her childhood that she shouldn't "rock the boat" and should keep small if she didn't want to cause trouble. She found it helpful to discuss the challenges of being assertive and speaking up for herself in our sessions and eventually began talking about it with friends and some trusted coworkers. Knowing she was not alone in these challenges in the workplace helped build her confidence that she could do something about it. She valued respect and recognition. These values served as pillars to overcome her fear of self-advocacy and speaking up. She pushed for an overdue raise. When she didn't get it, she left for a new job where she felt respected and recognized for her effort.

These are just a few of the success stories of the various people you met in this book. Across many of them, the commonality is that they dared to face the difficult feelings they had around perfectionism and were willing to do the work to understand it better and to transform their relationships to it in their lives.

The path forward: beyond perfectionism

In the pursuit of perfection and making others happy, somewhere along the way I lost sight of what it meant to truly live and feel fulfilled. I focused so much on the outcomes and success markers ascribed to me by others that I didn't know what I wanted for myself. Sometimes the pursuit of perfection felt like a thrill, don't get me wrong. It's not as though I didn't enjoy any aspects of the journey or the outcomes I achieved. I just didn't recognize the toll it took on me to have only focused on those external things for so long. And when I did recognize it, I knew something needed to change.

Change meant I had to face some difficult truths. I had to reckon with the loss of self-identity and a disconnect I felt from my values, interests, and passions for things outside of work and pleasing others. But it wasn't all doom and gloom. This reckoning also meant I had an opportunity to reconstruct something and build it up with things I wanted and valued. It also meant I could accept and embrace *all* of the parts of myself, including those at times I felt were hindrances to my happiness. I got to take ownership over my internal self – meaning getting back in touch with the stuff of dreams and real desires that lay beneath all of the trappings of productivity and "success."

Up to the point when I was asking things like "What is this for?" I had started to feel resentful towards the perfectionistic part in me. "Why do I have to be like this?" I blamed myself for feeling the way I did. But instead of blaming myself, I knew

I had to forgive myself, learn to accept and understand what that part was all about and the role it perhaps could still play in my life, albeit in some more constructive and healthy ways.

Like me, you may have spent the majority of your life trying to do your best at any cost. And like me, you may feel tired and confused about when you'll ever get some sort of "payoff" for all of this perfectionistic striving. It's a big step and a scary one to take when you even choose to pause and ask yourself how you're honestly feeling about your life. When you take stock of how you're feeling, it can be a wake-up call. Sometimes this wake-up call comes from external, uncontrollable factors such as a huge life event, loss, tragedy, or transition. Sometimes the wake-up call comes from something less dramatic but still very impactful – for instance, someone you listen to, read about, or speak to and they share a radically new perspective on how you might live your life. And sometimes the wake-up call just comes from that internal shift in you that says, "Enough is enough, something has got to change."

No matter what the cause of the wake-up call is, listen to that call and heed its message – that there's something new on the horizon for how you can think about life and take action towards it.

As I've said many times throughout this book, getting to acknowledge things for what they are is a powerful step. But it's also only one in a larger process. It's one important thing to acknowledge that we've been believing certain things that may no longer be true or serve us well. It's another to then take new information and find ways it can lead you in a better direction. And it's yet another to take action steps to practice the new things you've learned about yourself.

I invite you to go through this journey of building insight, relearning new ways of thinking and taking action. Do it unprepared. Do it slowly. Do it in small steps. Do it with the help of others.

In short, do it imperfectly. Imperfectly is better than doing nothing or doing more of the same that hasn't been helpful. And also because isn't that what we can expect of ourselves?

Useful resources

Brown, B. (2010) *The Gifts of Imperfection: Let go of who you think you're supposed to be and embrace who you are*. Center City, MN: Hazelden Publishing.

Brown, B. (2018) *Dare to Lead: Brave work. Tough conversations. Whole hearts*. London: Vermilion.

Burkeman, O. (2021) *Four Thousand Weeks: Time management for mortals* (First edition). New York: Farrar, Straus and Giroux.

Index